Contents

Acknowledgements

We are grateful for the time and effort put into this project by so many different people and organisations. First, we want to thank the people living in the residential homes for their willingness to try new things and their enthusiastic approach to all aspects of the work. We want to thank the staff and managers of the homes and of the Joseph Rowntree Housing Trust, City of York Community Services and East Riding Social Services. The work of the person-centred Planning Facilitators and Supported Employment workers was particularly influential – their positive and energetic approach made a real difference. The cooperation and commitment shown by so many people has been greatly appreciated.

1
Introduction

This book is based on a project set up to assist the Joseph Rowntree Housing Trust to improve the daytime opportunities open to people with learning difficulties and people with cerebral palsy living in their residential care homes. The project was an offshoot of the national Changing Days project and provided an opportunity to implement some of the findings and recommendations from that parent project. The work was led and managed by the King's Fund.

The book is about people who wanted things to be different in their lives and people who have been trying to assist them. It is about listening, planning, acting and problem-solving. It is about highs and lows, successes and struggles. It is about the experience of introducing new ways of improving people's lives and what we have learned on that journey – lessons we hope will be of benefit to other people trying to achieve change.

Background

In December 1994, the Changing Days project, funded by the Joseph Rowntree Foundation and the Gatsby Charitable Trust, began a three-year project to improve day opportunities for people with learning difficulties across the UK. The project worked with five development sites to support them in improving their services. It facilitated action learning sets and conferences to share lessons and examples of good practice, and produced publications (Wertheimer, 1996; Whittaker, 1999; McIntosh and Whittaker, 1998, 2000) which have influenced and helped large numbers of people working to improve day opportunities. In 1998 the project moved on to a second phase aiming to improve day opportunities for people who have complex disabilities.

Values

> ### The work of the Changing Days project was based on the belief that:
>
> - Disabled people have the ability and right to become full members of their local communities
>
> - Better daytime opportunities can be achieved by working in partnership with users, carers and staff in planning and shaping the future
>
> - The future for disabled people should be away from segregated day centres and building-based services towards being given support to participate in ordinary activities in the community
>
> - The emphasis should be on developing adult education, employment and meaningful leisure pursuits outside segregated services

Developments within the Joseph Rowntree Housing Trust

For some time the Joseph Rowntree Foundation has been keen to find ways of linking service delivery and practice to the recommendations from the research and development projects it commissions. A number of projects have been set up to demonstrate and learn from the practical implementation of new ideas and approaches.

The Foundation is well known as an organisation that commissions research and development projects and publishes reports in relation to community care. It is perhaps less well known that one arm of the Foundation, the Joseph Rowntree Housing Trust (JRHT), has provided residential services for people who have learning difficulties and/or physical disabilities since 1984. JRHT now supports 48 people living in four registered care homes, three within the York City Council area and one in the East Riding Council area. Therefore, the Foundation is in an ideal position to demonstrate new approaches through its own provision.

In 1995 JRHT evaluated its first care home and found that:

> "For the last 10 years a supportive environment has been carefully built ... it is obvious the residents feel secure and happy in that environment but a challenge for the future relates to the life chance opportunities which they have in the community. The challenge is to develop those opportunities and provide room for choices in the residents' daily lives."

The review made two particular recommendations:

● Consider ways of providing more opportunities for individual activities

● Investigate and discuss with local authorities the appropriateness of existing day care activities.

The JRHT Changing Days project was funded by the Joseph Rowntree Foundation to address the challenge of these recommendations. Work began in the autumn of 1997 and was extended in 1999 to include a supported employment initiative. The aim was to use the findings from the national project to develop best practice within its own organisation and, in the process, develop a better understanding of the issues involved.

Learning from the national project

Work during the first three years of the Changing Days project had clearly shown that "if there is going to be change then it must be informed centrally by the needs and wishes of those people who use or want a service". This must be the starting point of any initiative to improve opportunities for disabled men and women to lead lives of their own choosing. Along with this go a number of key ingredients needed for success:

Key ingredients

● Creating a commitment to change with a sense of urgency

● Capturing people's vision of how life could be

● Creating a culture of change and development

● Person-centred planning

● Understanding inclusion

● Moving from services to support for individual people

● Making it happen: having a game plan

The JRHT work has tried to put these principles into practice. A person-centred planning process built on the principles of Circles of Support (Wertheimer, 1995) has been the central tool in working towards these goals. Planning circles made up of family members, friends, neighbours and staff, were set up around individuals living in the homes. People chose who they wanted in their circle. The circles have helped individuals draw up a plan for their lives and then given active support to achieve specific goals.

The project has worked through some of the day-to-day challenges of putting ideas into practice around:
- person-centred planning;
- residential staff supporting people to do things from their home base;
- change management;
- partnership working across organisations;
- developing people's community involvement, social networks and natural support;
- supporting people to get and keep jobs;
- moving from group care to an individualised lifestyle chosen by the person.

Here is what some people have said about being involved in the work:

People living in the homes said:

"I look forward to planning what I'm going to do."

"I now go to watch football matches and have bought a season ticket."

"I have got a computer to help me speak more."

"I go line dancing now. I like it a lot."

"I do the collection at the church. I really like it."

"My circle is quite good. I get to meet people and do things."

"My friends come and visit me now."

"It makes me feel good."

Managers and staff said:

"It's opened our minds as carers: we're listening more."

"We've learnt to speak up for what people want."

"It's expanded our horizons – we can do it."

"The project has enabled parents and staff to appreciate the previously hidden abilities of residents and has helped them to fulfil people's goals and ambitions."

"Some good things seems to have opened up for all the people involved."

Recent initiatives in day opportunities

The 1990s have seen an improvement in the range of opportunities and experiences available to people with learning difficulties and disabled people more generally. Many local authority social services departments have conducted reviews of their day services for people with learning difficulties. The introduction of the 1995 Disability Discrimination Act has reinforced that people have a right to access public places and services and not to face discrimination. The New Deal employment initiative for disabled people has begun to offer targeted support so that people can actually get jobs and keep them. Progress has been made.

There have been numerous publications. In particular, the books from the Changing Days project have provided very practical guidance on how to develop new and better day opportunities, drawing on the experience of organisations around the UK. Another project funded by the Joseph Rowntree Foundation resulted in an important publication, *People, plans and possibilities* (Sanderson et al, 1997) that gives detailed guidance on person-centred planning.

The JRHT Changing Days project is able to add to this growing body of knowledge as it has approached the task from a different direction.

It has:

- been established within an **independent sector** organisation;

- supported a provider of **residential accommodation** to improve people's day opportunities and experiences;

- included **people with learning difficulties** *and* **disabled people** more generally;

- listened to residents' preferences and aspirations through **person-centred planning as a way of stimulating organisational change.**

Among many other things the project has shown how:

- an independent sector provider can lead the way and influence service developments more widely;

- a partnership between an independent sector provider and the local authority can lead to positive benefits for individuals;

- person-centred planning can lead to positive changes in people's lives, and is as helpful to disabled people as it is to people with learning difficulties;

- increased involvement of service users really does lead to increased empowerment;

- people's horizons expand when they see new opportunities opening up.

The project has helped us learn more about:

- how to put person-centred planning into practice;

- how to develop people's community involvement and social networks;

- the support and leadership that staff need;

- the resources that are needed to improve people's daytime opportunities and experiences.

2
Starting the journey

"It's very interesting – you plan things about your future."
(A resident)

Finding out what residents of the JRHT's homes wanted – their preferences, ambitions and dreams – had to be at the heart of the project.

The most important outcomes would be that people:

- achieved their hopes and wishes;

- had more individualised day opportunities;

- were more involved in their community;

- were less reliant on attendance at day centres.

The first step

Very early on in the project, a consultation day was held with residents and staff from the homes. This looked at three key questions:

- What is good about the way things are for people living in the homes right now?
- How could these things be changed to make them even better?
- What's the best that you could imagine?

People said things such as:
"It's boring."
"I'm enjoying it."
"It's dull."
"There are things I'm proud of."
"It's repetitive."

People wanted such things as:

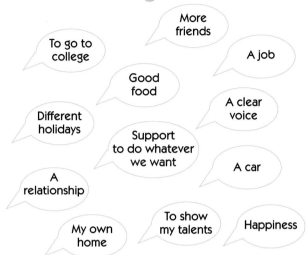

Figure 1: People living in the homes saw 'a good life' as ...

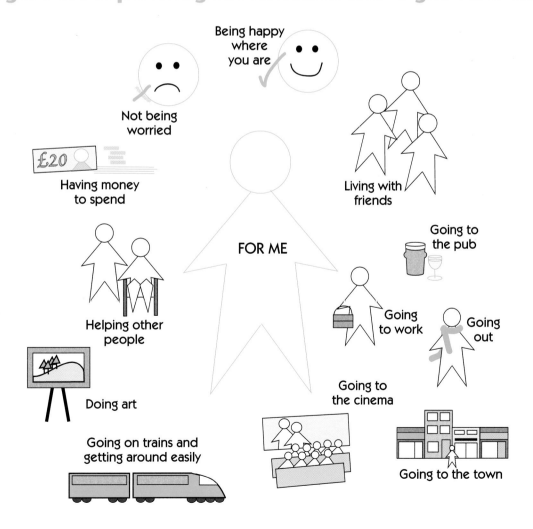

The picture at the beginning

People and places

When the project began in October 1997, there were 48 people living in the homes, 38 of whom were using local authority day services. Figure 2 shows the range of day services and opportunities people were using.

Figure 2: Range of day services and opportunities accessed by people in October 1997

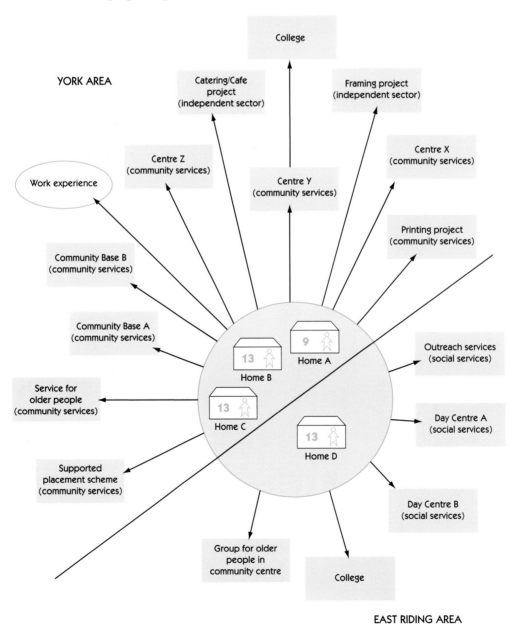

There was a striking difference in the range of provision in the two local authority areas reflecting, to some extent, the fact that York City Council is a small predominantly urban area and East Riding a larger predominantly rural area with significant distances between towns. The location of the four homes within the local authority areas is shown in Figure 3.

Figure 3: The four residential homes in relation to their respective local authority areas

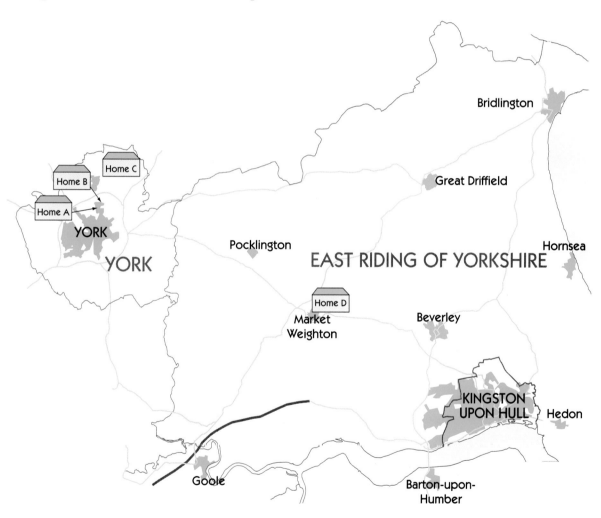

At the start of the project two people were in paid work, one in a supermarket and one at a Supported Placement Scheme workshop for disabled people, and two people were gaining work experience through unpaid jobs. Five others were on college courses, three of whom were approaching the end of long-term courses and were unsure about their next steps. Three people were not working or using any day services at all, two because of illness. Everyone else spent at least part of their week going to day service provision, with over half attending more than one type of opportunity each week.

People were spending varied amounts of time at home during the week. More staff were on duty in the early mornings and from mid-afternoon, reflecting the number of people out during the day.

Ages ranged from 20 to 67, with 12 people each in their 20s, 30s, 40s and 50s. Only two people were over 60, both women and both still using day service provision for at least part of the week. Ten people were under 25. No one in this age group was in work and three were coming to the end of college courses. There were 22 men and 26 women overall, with just one person from a minority ethnic background.

One of the homes was for people who have cerebral palsy. Of the nine people in this home only three were using local authority day services, and only part-time. Three people were on full-time college courses, two had paid employment and one was on a work experience placement. This was a different picture to the other three homes – all for people with learning difficulties.

The service

Days of change (McIntosh and Whittaker, 1998) highlighted six important things to do to make good things happen in people's lives:

- Persuading managers and other top people that it must be done
- Making sure that the changes are what disabled people want
- Organising services and the money that pays for them in a way that helps staff support people properly
- Making sure that each person has the chance to speak up for themselves and say what they want
- Supporting people a lot more to be involved in their local communities
- Having a plan to make all this happen

With these in mind there were some important factors about the service that the project needed to take into account:

- All the homes have been purpose-built within the last 15 years through partnerships between the JRHT and local organisations such as Mencap. Each has a Management Committee with representatives from the relevant partner organisations which meet quarterly. The Committees have a central role in the allocation of resources to the homes and in agreeing their service direction. The project would need to ensure that the Committees were informed and supportive.

- JRHT is a residential service provider but also aims to improve people's day opportunities. This meant that it needed to influence and involve a wide range of organisations who were already providing day services to residents. It was also clear that staff in the homes had little contact with staff in the day services and did not always know what people were actually doing during the day. A greater sharing of information and ideas, and working in partnership, was required.

- Generally speaking, staff and managers in the homes had little knowledge of current developments in services elsewhere so were having difficulty judging the quality of the service people were receiving within the JRHT. Few had received any training on the values and knowledge underpinning their work, nor help to develop skills to empower people living in the homes. Staff development would need to be central to the project.

- There was no standard individual planning system in operation across the homes and less than half the people had an annual review organised by their local authority. Not everyone had an opportunity to say what they thought of the services they were receiving or what they wanted in the future. Individual review meetings often focused on the skills that people needed to develop rather than the whole range of things they wanted to do and achieve in their lives. A different approach was needed that would give people an opportunity to talk about the things that mattered to them and then engage people in working together to make those things happen.

- Some of the service-wide systems operating across all the homes, while rooted in a caring approach and a concern to ensure people's security and comfort, were actually disempowering the people living and working in the homes. There were also some day-to-day practices that suggested staff needed support to treat people more individually, believing in each person's capacity and potential to make decisions and do things for themselves. There was a need for both staff and the organisation to develop risk management approaches and skills.

● Operational budgets and fee levels had been set with the expectation that people would be out of the home during the day using day services. For the majority of people the cost of their residential placement could be met fully from their benefits income and their local authority was not contributing. Securing more staff to support people during the day would require changes in the management of resources within the service and potentially, negotiations with the local authority about additional costs. This in turn would have implications for the local authorities' purchasing budgets. The project needed to support the organisations to identify ways of making their resources work best to support people to do the things they preferred to do.

● The capacity of the service to devote the time required to plan and lead the introduction of new approaches was limited. Day-to-day operational demands suggested that a project manager was needed to champion the changes and ensure that action happened. In the longer-term however, the project would need to ensure that managers in the service were taking on the leadership role to sustain the changes into the future.

A project plan

An initial project plan outlined a number of steps towards change, drawing on experience gained during the national Changing Days project.

Steps towards change

Create a values-base and culture shift through staff development and active leadership

▼

Find out people's preferences and goals through person-centred planning and consultation

▼

Support people to take more control over their lives through involvement and empowerment initiatives

▼

Build people's social networks and natural supports through planning circles and active community building

▼

Work towards inclusion and ordinary opportunities through community development and focused support

▼

Use the aggregate of person-centred plans to redesign services, and then implement changes

▼

Measure improvements by looking at changes in the quality of individuals' lives

The project identified four immediate priorities:

- To underpin the service development work with a set of shared principles and values

- To place the views, hopes and aspirations of people living in the homes at the heart of the initiative

- To create a sense of commitment and a desire to move forward collaboratively

- To provide active and focused leadership for the change effort

The project's path

A journey of any length often develops a life of its own – there are stops along the way, detours and enforced changes in the route. The project's journey similarly developed and changed during the two years. The key milestones and events are shown on the Project Path.

Figure 4: The project path

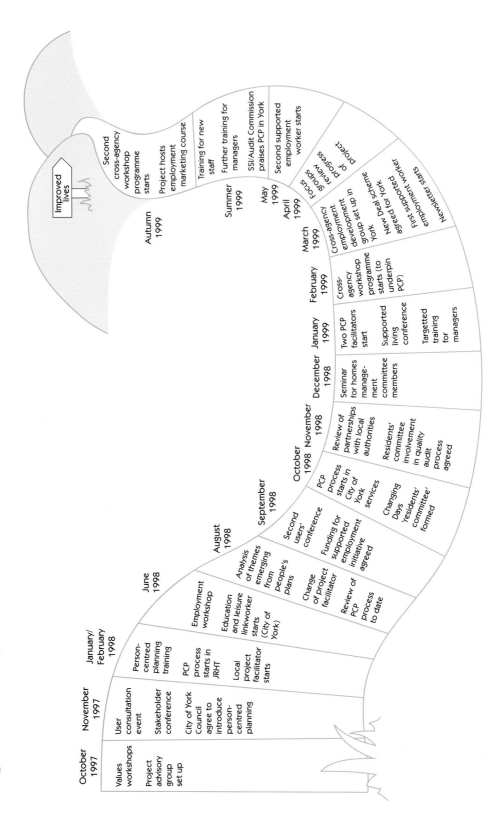

3
Creating a values base and culture shift

Other people see things and say 'why?'.... But I dream things and say 'why not?'
George Bernard Shaw

Changing the culture within an organisation is not easy. It involves a great deal of time, effort and commitment. It often takes much explanation, demonstration and reinforcement before people really understand and take on board new ideas and ways of working. In order to improve opportunities for people living in the JRHT homes, the project needed to influence and support a range of people to think and act differently:

- staff and managers in the homes and throughout the JRHT;
- members of the Homes Management Committees;
- staff and managers in the day services that people were using;
- members of people's families;
- people in the local community.

Locating local opportunities
Draw a map of the organisations and people in your area who could help improve people's opportunities for work, education, leisure and community involvement. Include all sorts of community-based organisations, not just the obvious 'service contacts'. These are all people you need to influence and get 'on board'.

It needed *sustained* effort throughout the project to embed common values and build a culture that would not only achieve change in people's lives but keep it going into the future.

A culture is needed which:

- sees it as essential to listen to and respect the views of service users;

- focuses on action that will change people's lives;

- encourages creative thinking;

- supports active problem solving and a 'we can do it' approach;

- encourages and values everyone's contribution;

- encourages staff to use their initiative and make decisions;

- promotes partnership working;

- looks beyond the organisation to create new opportunities;

- welcomes ideas and new developments;

- encourages people to reflect and learn from experience;

- encourages flexible use of resources to make things happen;

- has a clear commitment to equal opportunities;

- fosters a sense of 'ownership' in relation to the quality of the service.

A range of approaches was used to support the development of such a culture.

Staff development

- Workshops were held at the start to clarify values and develop a shared perspective

- Staff were introduced to person-centred planning by actually doing it with residents under the guidance of external trainers

- Project facilitators provided active support on the role and responsibilities of staff. Creative problem solving was encouraged

- Information folders about person-centred planning and developing day opportunities were placed in each home, and staff were regularly encouraged to read them

- JRHT staff participated alongside colleagues from the local authority and health trust in a comprehensive programme of training events. These included:
  - The national picture: Changing Days
  - Who's in Control? - Empowering People
  - Managing risks
  - Person-centred planning tools
  - Circles of Support
  - Building Community Connections & Involvement
  - An introduction to Supported Employment
  - Helping people learn
  - Quality matters
  - Supporting people with complex needs in community settings
  - Person-centred communication techniques

- New staff were introduced to the project and person-centred planning through sessions in each home using 'Dream Quest'[1]

- The induction programme was changed to reflect the new ways of working

[1] *Dream Quest: A game to teach the dynamic process of person-centred planning:* For more details contact Brian Remer, Monadnock Developmental Services, 640 Marlboro Street, Route 101, KEENE, New Hampshire, NH 03431, USA.

Management development

- Some senior staff were trained as person-centred planning facilitators; although they later passed this responsibility on, they gained a clear picture of the process and what needed to happen to make it work well

- Senior staff had sessions specifically focused on their role as leaders and managers in relation to person-centred planning

- Graphic facilitation training was given to senior staff to encourage creative approaches with their teams

- Senior staff took part in conferences on national developments on employment and supported living, alongside managers from partner agencies

Opportunities for staff involvement

- Staff and managers were regularly asked for feedback on the implementation of person-centred planning, and on the project more generally – responses were used to refocus the project plan

- Managers were involved in meetings with partner agencies to clarify roles and resolve operational problems

- Home support staff such as cooks and domestic staff were encouraged to join people's circles if invited

Information management

- Senior staff from partner agencies were involved in the Project Advisory Group; this ensured that information was disseminated and the project would influence developments more widely

- Seminars for members of the Homes Management Committees kept them up to date with progress and the changes in people's lives

- A two-monthly newsletter, including contributions by residents, let people know what had been happening for individuals. It was sent to staff, families, the residents committee, senior managers and the Homes Management Committees

- The Residents' Committee produced a booklet about their conference which was widely distributed, showing what people living in the homes had said about the developments so far and their hopes for the future

Modelling of different approaches

- Staff supporting people at the events organised by residents, observed the value placed on people's views and the responsibilities people carried during those days

- Staff and people living in the homes attended the training event on user empowerment in pairs; the workshop was run by a trainer with learning difficulties

- The graphic facilitation workshop encouraged senior staff to model a different way of recording; project staff also used graphics in their work

- Residents began the practice of being involved in the quality improvement process by undertaking an evaluation of one of the homes

Development of local champions

- Sessions for senior staff helped them think about what they could do to 'champion' new ways of working

- In recruiting two person-centred planning facilitators particular attention was paid to their commitment to the project's value base and whether they had a 'can do' approach

- Staff employed as facilitators and supported employment workers were given intensive training and supervision so that they could be positive models to others

- Members of the Residents' Committee were supported to develop as 'champions', speaking up for tenants and encouraging other residents to express their own views

- A partnership was established with York Community Services early on; the Director joined the project Advisory Group and operational links were cemented through secondment of a service manager to act as project facilitator. This very soon led to person-centred planning being adopted within City of York day services, with more local person-centred planning facilitators to champion the process

Developing a learning culture

The project needed to help the organisation develop a culture where people reflected on their practice and continually sought to improve it – a learning culture. Developing a learning culture within an organisation requires the following.

A focus on enabling and empowerment

A focus on enabling can be reinforced through a range of service management tools:
- The philosophy and objectives
- Policies
- Job descriptions
- Performance management criteria
- Supervision
- Training and mentoring
- On the job feedback
- Briefings

Messages that people are given through reading documents – the words used and the things that are said – help to create the culture. Being congratulated and thanked for doing things in ways that are wanted helps to cement it.

Paying attention to risk management

Staff often say that they worry about things going wrong; that they will be blamed and held responsible. They need to know what the boundaries are so that they have more confidence and feel supported in their work. This can be provided through operating an effective risk management policy. The policy needs to be supported in practice so that risk-management becomes an integral part of what staff do – it comes naturally and is automatically practised.

Risk management policy

A helpful policy emphasises:

- the benefits of new experiences and opportunities for people;
- that risk taking is part of daily life;
- that managing risks needs to be an integral part of everyday work;
- the need to ensure beneficial things happen as well as ensuring that negative things do not;
- the need to take an individualised approach – to look at risks specific to each person;
- the need to empower people so they can make their own informed choices;
- that decision making lies with the person and their planning circle;
- the need to manage risks for individuals in ways that do not compromise the lives of others;
- the importance of careful planning, monitoring, review and action learning.

Risk management is integral to the empowerment of disabled people. An organisation which aims to empower people through person-centred planning must support its staff to manage risk effectively.

Figure 4: Risk management

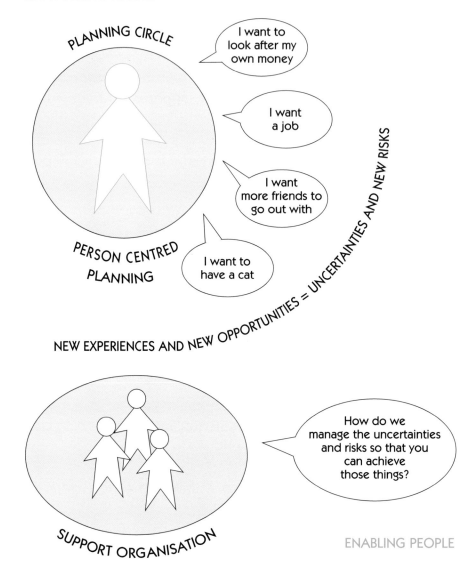

Leaders with a developmental approach

Good leaders:
- focus on improving outcomes for users and for staff;
- encourage staff to take responsibility and make decisions in their work;
- ensure they get information about new approaches, projects, debates;
- encourage people to try things out and implement new ideas;
- provide guidance, resources and support;
- are clear about boundaries and limits and where people can get help;
- encourage reflection and learning from practice;
- organise training and development opportunities;
- regularly and openly discuss performance with staff;
- ask questions such as: "What are you aiming to achieve?", "What did you learn?", "What would you do differently next time?", "How can we improve what we're doing?"
- use phrases such as: "Try a different way", "Good idea – write it up into a proposal for discussion", "Let's agree some goals and targets."

Developing a learning culture is not simply about giving people information and training. Ongoing management and support is key. It sometimes takes time for learning to happen.

> What is common practice is not always common sense, but we continue to do something until we are aware of that 'sense' ourselves. When we sense something deeper we start the process that culminates in a 'Eureka!'....
> (Turner, 1995)

4

Listening to people through person-centred planning

"One of the good things was about people listening to us when we were speaking up for ourselves."
(Residents)

Person-centred planning is a process that finds out what an individual wants to do with his/her life, helps the person decide on goals and then plans what action needs to be taken to achieve those goals. It is an ongoing process which means that the person can regularly set new goals as his/her skills and experience grow and ambitions change.

Person-centred planning has been developed in a number of different ways including personal futures planning, essential lifestyle planning and PATH (O'Brien, 1987; Mount et al, 1991; Smull and Harrison, 1992; Pearpoint et al, 1993).

The core principle in all of these methods is to look at the whole person rather than viewing them as a series of 'needs' – such as for residential, day or leisure services – and to consider all aspects of a person's life including friendships and relationships. The focus on each person as a unique individual is particularly important for people living in group residential provision where the wishes and needs of the many can overshadow that of an individual.

Person-centred planning:

- Puts the person – not the services – at the centre of the planning process

- Enables a person to take as much control of the process as possible

- Emphasises the importance of planning being done in ways that are 'right' for the individual and that enables him/her to participate

- Gives individuals a regular opportunity to talk about what they want in their lives

- Ensures that those who support the person regularly hear what he/she wants

- Brings together people who care about the person and harnesses their ideas, energy and commitment to make things happen for the individual

Person-centred planning is a tool that can result in people being able to:
- take part in activities that reflect their own preferences, interests, goals and ambitions;
- receive support geared to their particular needs;
- feel more positive about themselves and how they are being supported;
- take part in activities as equal citizens alongside other members of the community.

It can also mean that:
- services respond more flexibly and creatively to meet people's wishes and support needs;
- service planning and development is based on better information about what users want and need.

Circles of support

A circle of support is a group of people who meet together on a regular basis to help a person accomplish their personal goals in life. The members of a circle, who may include friends, family, neighbours, and interested members of the community are generally not paid to be there; they are involved because they care about the person and are committed to working with them to overcome obstacles and open doors to new opportunities. Service providers may also be involved, but the emphasis is on people who have natural ties to the focus person or who share common interests with them. (Wertheimer, 1995)

Ideally, a circle of support operates outside services. Being independent of services, it has the potential to take on an advocacy role for an individual, free of conflict of interest, which would be unlikely within a service framework.

The facets of circles of support which proved valuable in the Changing Days work were:
- getting people together right from the start, who are important to the person and who know him/her well, to share their knowledge and build up a positive picture of the person;
- involving friends, family and other 'unpaid' people;
- using informal settings for meetings and working in ways which suit the person;
- focusing on gifts and abilities;
- including people's hopes and dreams for the future.

The principles of person-centred planning are firmly embedded in circles of support. It was experience of the benefits which result from circles which influenced the Changing Days project to develop planning circles.

Planning circles

The work with the JRHT was based on each person having his/her own planning circle to help them work out what they wanted to achieve and how to go about it. Everyone chose to include in their circles staff who were working with them. Because the project was working with people living in residential homes – where their whole lives are directly influenced by an organisation – planning circles were helpful in drawing people *together* to work towards someone's goals both from within and outside of the service. This made an important contribution to changing the service culture.

Steps in the process

Giving the person information

Residents were asked if they wanted to think about how they could improve their lives. Not everyone chose to take part initially, but later on several people changed their minds as they saw others enjoying the planning circle meetings and realised that good things were beginning to happen. Making sure that an individual wants to be involved is an important principle in person-centred planning.

Forming the planning circle

It is important to explore in some detail who the person would like to ask to join their circle. This means spending time with the person and those close to him/her to identify contacts *beyond* services and immediate family. There may be people who were important to the person in the past who would be pleased to join the circle. Asking people to get involved is important. This part of the process should not be rushed.

Getting to know the person better

Circle members then need to build up a positive picture of the person as a unique individual with a unique life experience. This is a crucial part of the process. It links the person's past and present and gives clues about avenues to follow up in the future. It is helpful if the picture includes:

- How I communicate

- What has happened in my life

- The people in my life

- What I do now, where I do it and who with

- The support I need

- What I enjoy – what I don't enjoy

- What I have control over in my life

- My talents and interests

- My dreams and ambitions

It is important to ask people about things they have enjoyed in the past. Many people stop doing things because of changes in their support rather than because they wanted to.

> When Conrad was asked by his planning circle if there was anything he used to do and enjoy that he doesn't do any longer he told people about his interest in rugby. He used to play himself and help young children with their training. Although no one in his circle had an interest in rugby someone knew someone who did. This contact led to Conrad being linked with the person who coaches young children in the nearby town, and his interest in rugby was rekindled.

Conrad meeting with his planning circle

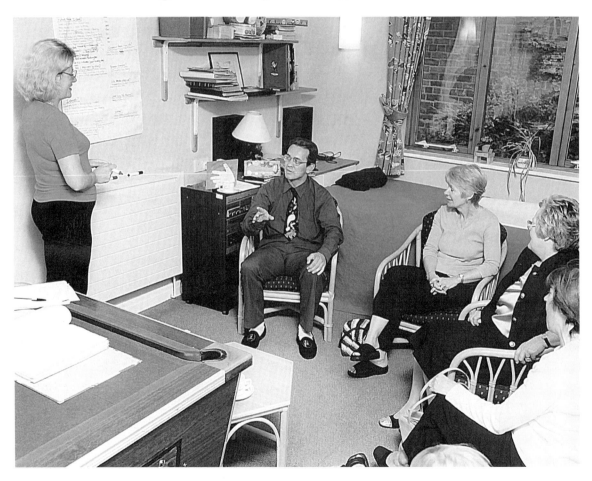

This part of the process is ongoing: the picture builds up as the person tries new opportunities and as the circle shares more information. It is important to record it so that it is not lost for the future.

> During one of her early planning circle meetings, Michelle told people she wanted to spend time each day lying on the floor – it helps her to feel comfortable. Her mother was surprised to hear that the care staff did not know about this as Michelle was used to doing it when at home.

Helping the person to 'dream for the future' and develop a plan

The following areas give planning circles a focus for goal setting and action planning. The list can be added to and built on over time.

- Current activities the person enjoys and wants to continue

- Activities the person used to enjoy and might like to take up again

- New activities he/she would like to try or to learn

- Areas of their life where they would like more choice and control

- Relationships, friendships and social circle

- Hopes, dreams and ambitions

Agreeing and prioritising goals

Some people find it difficult at first to identify what they would like to do or achieve. Circle members too, unused to the process or the opportunity to think creatively, can find it difficult to help the person with new suggestions: goals may seem disappointingly small and unimaginative. In this case, goals that focus on trying things out can be helpful. To make early achievements more likely it helps to set short, medium and longer-term goals and no more than five goals at any one time. People's horizons expand the more often they meet together and achieve more goals together, so keeping the circles going is important.

Agreeing the support needed

Each person is probably already receiving support for some basic core needs. These need to be taken into account when discussing the person's new goals and what additional support might be needed. Where someone has more complex needs it is helpful to ask whether they would be prevented from, or hampered in achieving their goal if any of their basic support needs weren't met. In many cases the answer will be 'yes' so the planning circle needs to make sure that the person receives support with those needs.

Planning action

It is crucial that the planning circle concentrates on how to achieve the person's goals in ways that develop more ordinary life patterns, that is, doing things alongside non-disabled people in ordinary community settings where there will be more opportunities to make friendships and take on valued roles. Many planning circles need support to move away from service-led options and to focus on community solutions.

A creative community-focused action plan

One of Martin's goals is to play snooker more often – preferably every Wednesday night.

Our action plan

- Martin, with Pete's support, will find out about joining the local snooker club or the social club and choose which one he wants to join

- Martin will go to the Building Society with Ann to withdraw the money to pay for his membership

- Susan will make sure Pete is on duty on Wednesday evenings so he can go with Martin to the club for the first four weeks

- Pete will try to find someone at the club who will play snooker with Martin regularly and help him improve his game

---

Keeping in contact, checking progress and solving problems

Making things happen can be far from straightforward. Circle members who have taken on tasks as part of the action plan need regular support and encouragement. Developing creative problem-solving skills is important and stressing the value of the work helps to keep people positive and motivated.

Celebrating success and agreeing new goals

Person-centred planning is a process, not a one-off exercise. Our priorities and ambitions can change over time, sometimes fairly rapidly as we discover our own potential and learn about new opportunities. It is essential that the person keeps in regular contact with members of their planning circle so that they can celebrate achievements, work out a different approach if progress is slow and plan new goals.

Frequency of meetings

How often the planning circle meets should be decided by the person with his/her circle members. Meeting more frequently at the beginning – say not less than once a month – is important to establish the group and get people working together well. It can be difficult for members to commit themselves to regular meetings but it does pay off. Circles that meet together more often achieve goals more quickly. Not every meeting has to include 'business'. There may not be much to report with regard to the circle's action plan but that does not mean the circle should not meet. Having a good time socially deepens friendships and strengthens the person's 'ties and connections'.

Later on, when the circle – and therefore the person's social/support network – is well established, meetings in the more formal sense of the word may naturally become less frequent. Circles may still meet together for group socialising or to help with a particularly difficult problem, but contact may also be through 'phone calls, one-to-one meetings, or sending notes. The important thing is that progress towards a person's goals is maintained and in a way which suits the individual. Keeping circle members involved is about good liaison, information and support, but it is also about commitment to the person as a friend.

Person-centred planning is more than meetings

Paula does not like the idea of meetings but said she'd like to have a coffee morning to talk about things. She decided who to invite and a planning circle was born. Initial goals were relatively small, but Paula has set the pace and enjoys her coffee mornings because she is in control of them.

Circle membership

Many planning circles begin with quite small numbers. This is not necessarily a bad thing but it can be very disappointing for the person concerned, if people send apologies or simply don't turn up, particularly when it is the first meeting. Following-up and encouraging people to take part in a person's planning circle is really important. Large numbers are not necessary, but the more people there are in the 'core' of regular attendees, the more people there are to share tasks resulting from the action plan and to support each other and the disabled person generally.

> "We want to improve the meetings and get more friends and outside people involved in them."
> Changing Days Residents' Committee Conference Report, 1998

Facilitating planning circles

Good organisation and facilitation of planning circle meetings is essential. At one of their conferences, people living in the homes showed how much this mattered to them.

> "Some of us had meetings that were too long and people didn't turn up on time."

Planning circles need someone who will take on a facilitation role to ensure that:
- the person is supported to make arrangements for the circle meetings;
- the person's needs and wishes remain the central focus;
- planning is done in ways which involve and empower the person;
- everyone's views are heard and valued, and differences of opinion are mediated;
- goals are agreed and action is planned;
- action agreed is not governed by service-led options and constraints;
- members of the circle receive support and encouragement to stay involved.

Facilitating planning circle meetings in a person-centred way is a skilled task. People need to be able to:
- explain in plain language what it's all about;
- create openings for the person to take the lead;
- pick up non-verbal clues that the person may be unhappy about what's being said, or is losing interest or getting tired;
- help people feel relaxed, comfortable and able to have fun while also keeping the discussion moving forward;
- handle differences between people in ways which build consensus;
- ensure that the goals set really do reflect what the person wants;

- challenge circle members to think beyond existing services when considering how to achieve goals;
- ensure that goals and action plans agreed are feasible within the time that circle members are able to give, while still keeping momentum going;
- Record decisions and plans in ways that mean something to everyone present.

Practical ways to ensure that circle meetings are 'person-centred'

- Help the person to arrange the seating and decide who they want to sit next to. If the person can't tell you, find out from others where the person feels comfortable and who they seem most at ease with
- Find out how often the person would like a break and if they want to stay with their circle for all or only part of the meeting
- Support the person to welcome their circle members as they arrive
- Make sure that refreshments are available and involve the person in preparing and serving them
- Support the person to set some ground rules for the circle – things that will help make it a good experience for the individual and the circle members
- Identify how the person can be actively involved in the discussions. For example, using pictures to make choices, drawing and writing notes, time-keeping, teaching circle members any signs or symbols the person uses
- Ask people to bring photographs to help build up the picture of the person's life and as part of the record of the discussion
- Use objects as visual prompts – for example, things they have made, important possessions, medals and certificates
- Draw lots of pictures to illustrate the discussion, and have a 'library' of pictures of ordinary objects and activities that can be used to generate ideas and discussion
- Avoid jargon! Use ordinary words that mean something to the person

---

It takes time and encouragement for someone to gain the confidence to take the lead in talking and planning about themselves. People need support to make their planning circle meetings their own. This is also likely to mean helping other people to give up some of their power and control.

At his third circle meeting Geoffrey decided to take charge of writing information on the flipchart paper. He also decided he would like to meet more often with his planning circle, but for a shorter time. When his next meeting was due he wrote his own invitation letters and sent them out. He is now much more in control of the process.

At his third meeting Andy decided he wanted to have a say in where people sat so he wrote out name labels and put them on the seats he wanted people to sit in.

Jamie didn't enjoy his first circle meeting very much and it was well over a year before he decided he would try again. At the second meeting of his planning circle he decided to set some rules that he wanted people to follow. It helped.

Who should facilitate planning circles?

Ideally, it should be the person whose circle it is, with support if they need it. The reality is that some disabled people will be able to take on the role fairly quickly but many will need long-term support. Ideally too, the facilitator should be independent – able to be 'on the side' of the focus person, free of any conflict of interest. However, where planning circles are initiated within a service as part of its person-centred planning system, it is likely that facilitators – in the early stages at least – will be keyworkers or other members of staff. It is crucial, therefore, that everyone involved with the planning circles understands the importance of independent facilitation and keeps working towards that goal. 'Paid' facilitators should always be working towards handing over the role to the person him/herself or to some other member of the circle. It can help if the facilitator shares the role with another circle member, or perhaps supports two circle members to share the role.

It is important too, that the circle lets the person have opportunities to take a lead. For disabled people, disempowered throughout their lives, this is a key issue. If circle members are actually trying to get the person to do what *they* want him/her to do, the person is unlikely to develop the skills needed to be able to take the lead and will continue to need the support of the facilitator.

At the start of the project 11 people were trained to facilitate planning circles for people living in the homes. All were senior staff or managers from the homes and from local day services. After nine months it became clear that these staff were having great difficulty in keeping the process going. Pressures on time because of their other work responsibilities and 'conflict of interest' issues arising because of their position within services, made it extremely difficult for them to maintain the person-centred principles and meet the objectives of the planning circles.

Independent facilitators

A decision was made to create two half-time posts with a specific remit to facilitate the planning circles. The staff were employed by the JRHT but were independent of the homes. They were given close supervision and support by project staff.

Being one step removed from the homes, the two facilitators did not experience the same conflict of interest as staff in the homes might well do, for example when liaising with parents and family members, or with managers. They could hold more firmly to the principle that the person should be the driving force in the planning process, without jeopardising working relationships in the homes. For example, when a difficulty arose between a person and their parent over setting a date for a planning circle meeting, the facilitator was able to support the person's wishes and the meeting went ahead on the date the person had chosen.

> A mother did not want her daughter to do voluntary work in a particular charity shop. The facilitator gave her more information and encouraged her to visit the people who ran the shop. This reassured her that it would be alright.

Once the facilitators were in post the quality of the planning improved and it became a more satisfying experience for everyone involved. The investment of time and funds soon resulted in more people achieving things they wanted to do. This suggests that effective facilitation is more likely if it is a significant part of a person's job. It also means that circle members' energy and commitment are more effectively harnessed for the benefit of the individual.

Key requirements for an effective facilitator

- Independence from direct service provision

- Absence of personal control over the individual

- Ability to give the time needed to ensure that the planning process happens and is person-centred

- The ability to do the things listed on **page 38**

When reviewing the project, staff made a number of comments about facilitation:

> "Bring outside facilitators in early. With managers facilitating it's too much like a formal meeting."

> "Employing two facilitators has worked well. It's been very positive."

> "Having the facilitators has been the most useful thing."

Who else needs to be involved?

Person-centred planning is not about passing all the responsibility to the planning circle and its facilitator. The support of other people, both in and outside services, is vital in order to achieve people's goals.

Keyworkers

If the person-centred planning is being driven by a service, the role of keyworkers is very important. It is highly likely that an individual will invite his/her keyworker to join their circle. They will be in an ideal position to offer the person direct support, for example with preparing and presenting information about their life to share with their planning circle.

Other things that the keyworker can do are:

- explain to the person what the planning circle is all about;
- help him/her to work out who to invite to join their circle and to send out invitations;
- support the person to take things to their planning circle meeting;
- make sure the person speaks up and plays an active part in the circle meeting and is listened to by the circle members;
- help the person decide which ambition/dream/goal they want to work on first;
- support the person to go through the record of their goals and action plans and keep motivated to achieve them;
- keep a running list of all the goals a person has achieved;
- keep circle members informed about progress;
- organise a 'celebration' when someone has achieved a goal.

Managers

Managers are also critical to the success of person-centred planning.

Staff identified the following ways in which managers can support and show their commitment to the process:

- Be very person-centred in your day-to-day work
- Ensure that keyworkers are supporting people to prepare for their planning circle meetings and help them think creatively about how to do this
- Be aware of the goals and plans a person has chosen
- Make sure the goals are not just about one-off trips and events but are about sustained change
- Make sure that people can do things more than once – that it keeps happening
- Support the people who are trying to make the goals happen – for example, give keyworkers time to take the necessary action
- Encourage staff to do the things they said they would do
- Enable staff to make decisions and take responsibility for moving things forward
- Support staff to identify opportunities to develop 'natural supports' for the person
- Show a real interest in how things are progressing
- Ask about person-centred plans in staff supervision sessions and staff meetings
- Help people with problem-solving
- Use resources flexibly and creatively, especially staffing
- Make sure the person's action plan is not just about being slotted into an existing service
- Use your links and contacts to make things happen
- Make sure that results are achieved
- Say thank you and well done when someone's actions have led to a person achieving a goal
- Celebrate achievements
- Be a champion!

Ancillary staff

Previously the Trust had not encouraged ancillary support staff to do things with residents on a more social level outside their working hours. When person-centred planning was first introduced this had stopped some ancillary staff from volunteering their time. As the process began to affect the culture of the organisation, the contribution of ancillary staff was welcomed and encouraged.

Heather was very keen to learn to cook for herself but the home she lived in employed a cook who usually prepared the residents' meals. When the cook heard about Heather's wish she offered to help her do some cooking and it has now become a regular date.

Figure 5: The JRHT process in a nutshell

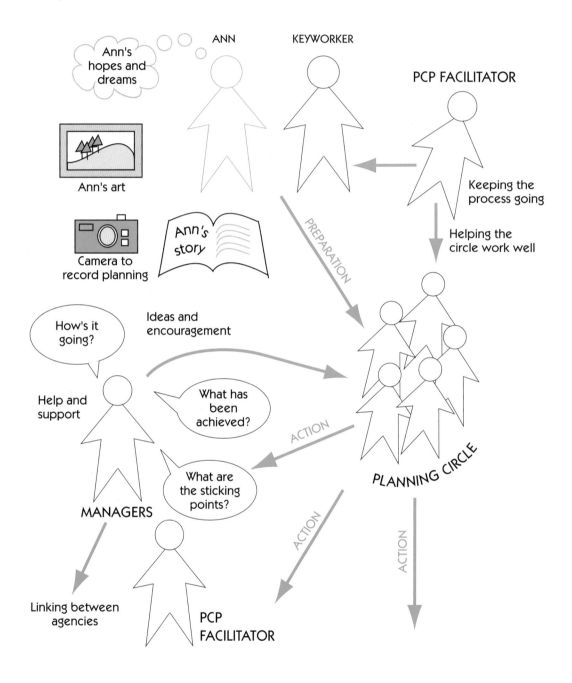

There are a number of things that need to be done to make a person-centred planning process work well within an organisation, and more importantly, work well for the individual. It is crucial that people at all levels in an organisation understand that they have a role to play.

Documenting the planning process

Part of the process of person-centred planning is making sure that the person has their own record of the planning that is meaningful. As well as the written word, this could involve using braille, audio-tape, video, photos, pictures, graphics and symbols. Part of the record needs to be in a form suitable to use as a reminder to circle members of the goals and plans, and to keep centrally to inform service planning.

A loose-leaf system provides flexibility in filing and updating a variety of material and enables particular pages or sections to be easily copied and held elsewhere if necessary. This might apply to information needed for service planning or confidential personal information. This method avoids unnecessary duplication while still maintaining the record as something the person him/herself 'owns' and uses.

It is important to keep in mind that both types of information are important and to avoid the danger of only producing the textual information required by the organisation.

The national Changing Days project has produced a personal planning handbook which can be used as the basis for documenting the planning process. It is published as part of the book *Unlocking the future* (McIntosh and Whittaker, 2000).

Andy showing people the poster about his life

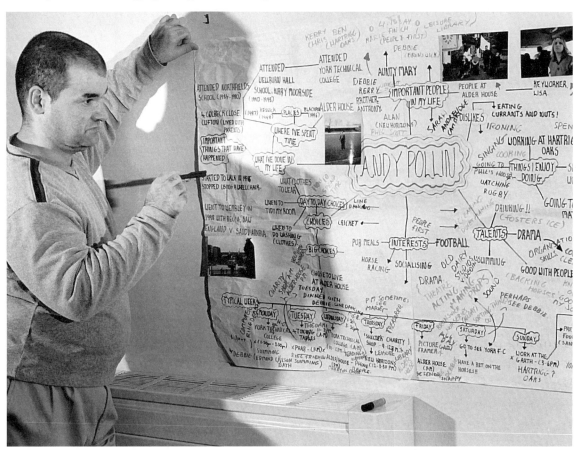

The role of families in person-centred planning

It is of course crucial that families are involved in the planning process if the person wants this. Experience during the national Changing Days project revealed a number of factors that seemed to make a positive difference in involving parents and family members. The York work reinforced that experience as the quotes show:

● Focusing on the individual as a person with gifts and abilities, rather than as someone with deficits and needs. Staying focused on positive outcomes for the person.

"I've learned more about my son and his views in the last two hours than I have in the last 27 years."

One man's relatives found out through his circle meeting that he used makaton: "We thought he was playing charades."

- Focusing strongly on relationships, social networks and community activities rather than services: it enabled 'person-centred' thinking rather than 'service' thinking.

- Informality and friendliness.

  "It felt more equal."
  "I've never been to anything like this before." (A resident's cousin)

- The paperwork is fun and user-friendly – not a matter of filling in pages of detailed forms.

- Parents and staff valued the opportunity of spending more time than usual getting to know people better and learning more through the circle meetings.

  "This is the first time I have felt that people are really listening to X and me."

A guiding principle of person-centred planning is that the focus person's views come first. However, there are times when other people have a different view of what's best for him or her and conflict arises. For disabled adults this conflict is often with their parent(s) and often centres around the parents' genuine fears about risks that their son or daughter may face. Because planning circles bring a range of people together who care about the person, it is more likely that a positive way forward will be found which both reassures and supports the parents but also enables the individual to progress towards his/her goal.

> During a circle meeting it became very clear that Barry wasn't enjoying a class he was attending and wanted to stop going. His nearest relative was not at all happy with the idea. The situation was resolved when another relative spoke up in support of the person's own wishes and suggested another way forward.

Strengthening the planning circle

Organisations and their staff are regularly subject to development and change. People come and go and this can seriously affect the continuity of services and support to the people using the service. This is one very good reason for deliberately working to build the strength of planning circles because they have the potential to overcome this problem. Since they aim to be made up largely of ordinary citizens and not staff – people paid to be there – they should not be subject to change to such a great extent.

Much effort needs to be put into involving people outside services if we are to realise the full benefit which can be gained through the planning circle process and thus achieve better quality lives for the people they support.

5
Empowering people

"The meetings help us to think and listen."
(A resident)

"I can speak my mind."
(A resident)

The whole of the Changing Days work was based on the principle of putting disabled individuals at the centre of services, enabling them to develop a lifestyle of their choice and become valued citizens alongside other members of the community. Essentially, this was done on two levels – empowering people as individuals and through working together as a group.

On the individual level, each person was helped to speak up for themselves and work out an action plan for their lives through their planning circle. The way this was done and many of the stories about how this changed people's lives is detailed in other chapters.

This chapter talks mainly about how the project sought to empower people through helping them to work together and how services can contribute to empowering people through the way it involves them in various service-related opportunities.

Working in partnership with users

A strong theme running through the national Changing Days project has been involving service users themselves, working alongside professionals to change services. User groups were set up in all the development sites and achieved a variety of successes in influencing the development of services (Wertheimer, 1996; Whittaker, 1999; McIntosh and Whittaker, 1998, 2000). In all the sites there was already a tradition of encouraging self-advocacy and enabling people to speak up for themselves. In some sites it was firmly established. For example, in Newham there was a People First group that was able to take a leading role in the Changing Days work there. In other sites, Changing Days provided the catalyst for re-establishing and strengthening previous work. This happened in Hereford and Knowsley where the user groups set up during the project have become the local voice for people with learning difficulties.

The situation in York

Although JRHT residents were encouraged to speak up for themselves to a certain extent, this was mainly in the context of house meetings held to discuss holidays and issues relating to the running of their home. Their experience of active, independent self-advocacy was thus very limited. Managers were keen to give people the opportunity to develop this area of their lives and fully supported the principle of working with users.

The work in York began with a user consultation day. People from the homes talked about their current lives and what they wanted to do in the future. This was not only an important starting point for the project's work generally but set the scene for introducing the idea of forming a group which would speak up for all the people in the homes.

The Changing Days Residents' Committee

A small committee of representatives was set up and met regularly. The group chose their own name and elected officers. At the time of writing they had achieved a great deal in the 18 months of their existence.

Their achievements include:
- organising two residents' conferences;
- producing conference reports;
- taking part in the JRHT's quality audit by checking the services at one of the homes;
- taking part in staff training workshops.

Committee members were proud of:
- "Being on the committee."
- "Doing reports."
- "Organising our own conference in York."
- "Helping to chair the London Changing Days conference."
- "Speaking up more."

Various members of the committee took on leadership roles in a number of different ways:
- contributing as a speaker at a Project Advisory meeting;
- making a presentation at a seminar for Management Committee members;
- chairing their own conferences and assisting with chairing a national Changing Days user conference;

- writing to and meeting with the service director to discuss funding and other matters.

The aims of the committee

- To solve residents' problems

- To raise money for things people wanted to do

- To help people to learn things

- To work with other speaking up groups

- To ask questions and get answers

Formalising the Changing Days residents' group

The group has now held its first AGM and elected an enlarged committee. It agreed a constitution and opened a bank account which enabled it to apply for funding from a national grant-making body. The formalising of the residents' group was an important step. It helped everyone become clearer about what they were there for and what they could do.

Spreading the word about achievements

The written word is a powerful way of telling other people about your achievements and encouraging others to do the same.

The JRHT residents produced a report of their conference that was widely distributed within the organisation. This demonstrated the value attached to that conference and the importance of people speaking up for themselves.

Residents also contributed to the Changing Days newsletter, writing their own stories about their achievements through their planning circles.

Involvement in quality audit process

Carrying out an evaluation of one of the homes was a significant step forward for the committee. It involved:

- talking about what it means to check a service, why service users get involved and how other people have done it;

- thinking about what makes a good home life and developing a questionnaire which they felt was right for them;
- training on how to interview people and ask questions;
- interviewing people individually and in a group;
- discussing the results and writing a report.

The committee made the following comments about being involved:

"It's a good idea because we talked to residents and asked questions. If you don't ask questions you don't learn. We were trying to learn what they do in the home."

"I enjoyed meeting people. I liked working on helping people answer the questions."

"I felt confident in doing the task. I felt a bit nervous about what to say."

"I've liked doing it."

By involving residents in checking their own services, JRHT demonstrated its commitment to the principle of working in partnership with the people it serves. The work of the group went beyond consultation, to real involvement. Group members made judgements about the quality of the service that they visited, and their recommendations were viewed as important by the organisation. Several things changed in the home they visited because of their comments.

Other opportunities

JRHT residents had a number of other opportunities to learn more about speaking up for themselves and broaden their horizons. For example, they took part in conferences and workshops organised during the project on supported employment, supported living and user empowerment. On these occasions, other disabled people leading workshops and talking about their lives were valuable role models.

As a result of being involved with the supported living conference, people living in one of the homes set out to learn more about different housing options. They invited people who lived in flats to come and talk to them and visited people living in different types of housing. Getting information in this way helped expand their horizons and see that other lifestyles are possible.

Inclusiveness

At a recent seminar, a young black woman with learning difficulties stressed that:

"If you are from an ethnic minority and have a learning difficulty and complex needs – double, double, double whammy."

Empowering disabled people means taking into account ways in which individuals face double or triple levels of disadvantage or discrimination – because of their ethnicity, gender, age, sexual orientation or complex needs.

Taking positive action

The project tried to ensure that there was an inclusive approach that empowered people most at risk of being marginalised. Person-centred planning achieves this very effectively because of its individualised focus, but it was still important to stop and reflect, regularly, whether the outcomes being achieved with people who have more complex needs were comparable to those achieved with others.

With the residents' committee it was important that everyone had a role and could make a contribution to the running of the meetings, from chairing the meeting to making drinks or handing out papers.

> Becca, the only black resident in any of the homes, was keen to join the committee. This gave her the opportunity to go to a national users' conference where she met other black people who were speaking up for themselves. This was something that she clearly enjoyed and valued.

> People who use services in Oldham came to the residents' group AGM to talk about their experience of person-centred planning. Afterwards members of the committee commented that information about a man with very complex needs was what they found most interesting.

Conclusion

JRHT residents achieved much during the short life of the project, both as individuals and in their work as a group. However, supporting people to speak up for themselves and each other is very time-consuming, particularly in the early stages when people are still developing the confidence and skills which will enable them to take more control later on.

Most groups need and benefit from:

- Consistent, hands-on support, preferably from an independent facilitator

- Resources – for example, money, a place to meet, an office or 'space' which is for the group's use

- Being within a culture which values and actively encourages people to speak up for themselves and take more control

- Support from managers and others in a position to 'champion' their cause

- Time to develop at their own pace. This includes time to socialise and get to know each other away from the formality of meetings

- Documents such as a constitution and set of rules in a format which suits the needs of the group and enables people to understand the necessary formal aspects of running a group

The Changing Days project was a catalyst in enabling people to feel more empowered and begin to develop the skills necessary to work together to change their own lives and be able to influence change in the lives of their friends.

An effective user involvement strategy

In a service with effective user involvement we would see at the strategic level:

- Regular contact with users by people at the top – example, managers, planners, policy makers, councillors

- Users on committees and sub-groups with appropriate support

- Parallel user groups with negotiating power and a clear process for joint working with staff/professional groups

- A budget for user involvement seen as essential and non-negotiable – part of mainstream funding, not just an 'add-on' offered when there is some spare money

- Users involved in monitoring and evaluation on an on-going basis

- User involvement written into contracts. Providers should be able to demonstrate how they enable the voice of users to be heard and give examples of how users influence the way their service operates

In a service with effective user involvement we would see at the practice level:

- Users centrally involved in all aspects of planning about their lives

- People choosing their own support workers, including hiring and managing their own workers with help from direct payment legislation

- An effective person-centred planning process which ensures that people's views are heard by planners

- An easy to use and well-used complaints procedure

- Active groups and committees in homes, day services and clubs, which can demonstrate that users are sharing power and control with professionals

- Groups specifically for people from minority ethnic groups to provide opportunities to discuss issues of particular relevance to their cultural group

- A user involvement officer – preferably an independent person

- A member of staff whose job is to spend at least part of their time supporting people specifically in 'user involvement' activities, for example, people need support not only to get meetings and take part in them but support later when they report back to their peers and staff

- Joint training as a regular practice – users and staff training together and users training staff

- Users involved in the appointment of staff

- People working in health, social services and education offices (paid, unpaid, full time, part time) – all statutory departments would have a proactive policy towards this end

- User-friendly, accessible information in different languages and formats

- Advocacy services

6
Listening to people: implications for services

"I now go to watch football matches and have bought a season ticket."
(A resident)

"My friends come and visit me now."
(A resident)

Person-centred planning must be linked to service planning, development and monitoring in order to achieve services that *can* and *do* support individuals in their chosen lifestyle. This presents a challenge to service providers, particularly where the service provision is still organised around groups.

Let's do it!
Major service reorganisation may be needed in the longer-term, but there is a lot that can be done immediately.

Here are some questions for managers to consider:

- How can you organise the time of existing staff differently?

- What public services or facilities are already there that the person could join or use?

- Can you borrow equipment?

- Are people getting all the income they are eligible for?

- Who could you involve from *beyond* services?

- How could you support people to directly ask services for more resources – self-advocacy?

Some of these are discussed in this and the next two chapters.

What is needed most is a positive 'let's do it' approach – encouraging people to try options, think widely and problem solve together. It makes all the difference.

Using information from person-centred planning

It is important to:

- Collate information
- Analyse it
- Use it

The project set up a central database containing information from everyone's planning.

We found it helpful to focus on people's aspirations in six main areas:

- Employment/work
- Leisure
- Learning
- Control/autonomy
- People/relationships
- Accommodation

The database also collated people's support needs in relation to five areas:

- Daily living and personal care
- Travelling
- Communication
- New opportunities
- Health

It is important to recognise that people's goals and wishes change and develop over time. This was quite marked in the 18 months after person-centred planning was introduced within the Housing Trust. So, collecting and analysing information is not a one-off activity. It needs to be done at set intervals to really capture what people want and to be useful for service planning. The goalposts do change!

Collating and analysing information in this way takes time. It is more aligned with research than service delivery and it is essential that it is done by people with the necessary knowledge, skills and allocated time.

Consultations with people using services around the UK indicate that there are five central themes for change which were echoed by people living in the Housing Trust homes. Services need to develop opportunities and support for people to do the following.

Find and keep work

More than half the people involved in the project said that they would like to get a job. Almost all wanted it to be part-time and paid, although the possible effect on their benefits was a genuine worry.

Take part in more varied and ordinary leisure pursuits

Everyone wanted to do more and/or different leisure pursuits. Many of these usually take place in the evenings and at weekends like watching the local football team and going to RNLI meetings.

Learn more and increase their independence

Around half the people identified particular things they wanted to learn or skills they wanted to improve. Some of these were leisure focused, some were about general life skills. Some people wanted to live more independently.

Have greater control over their life

Initially few people talked about wanting more control over aspects of their lives – but this changed as time went on. After 18 months more than half had identified specific areas such as who they lived with, shopping, choice of holidays, or their weekly routine.

Develop their friendships and relationships

Several people said they wanted to make new friends. Others said they wanted to have someone to go out with. Many wanted to see relatives and friends they hadn't seen for some time.

This is what people want. The rest of this chapter examines some of the ways that services can support people to achieve the first four of these. The fifth area – friendships and relationships – is discussed in Chapter 7.

Supporting people to find and keep work

Disabled people face discrimination and disadvantage when trying to secure work. Since 1999 the implementation of specific employment-related provisions in the 1995 Disability Discrimination Act has begun to address this issue with employers. However, the reality is that many of the past government-led initiatives have failed disabled people who need systematic and often sustained support to find and keep a job in an ordinary workplace.

Two developments in the UK have addressed this – the setting up of supported employment agencies and the creation of small (usually subsidised) businesses with specific objectives to employ disabled people – often organised as cooperatives or 'social firms'.

What is 'supported employment'?

There is often confusion about supported employment because the term is used in Britain to mean two different things. Here we are using it to describe the process of supporting a person – in whatever way and for as long as they need – to get and keep a job in an ordinary work setting which matches their individual preferences and talents, and which will bring with it the full benefits of employment.

The Association for Supported Employment

The Association for Supported Employment (AfSE) encourages and promotes the development of supported employment in the UK. It has a membership of more than 200 organisations and individuals. The Association actively seeks to influence government and the development of national policy and practice.

AfSE can be contacted at:
Pennine View, Gamblesby, Penrith, CA10 1HR
Website: http://www.afse.org.uk
Email: afsc@Onyxnet.co.uk

Social firms

A social firm is a business or commercial company which has explicit social objectives, setting out to employ a significant proportion of disabled people at the going market rate for the job. Social firms are often run as cooperatives.

For more information on cooperatives contact:
ICOM, Vasselli House, Leeds,
Telephone: 01532 461737
See also: Grove, B. et al (1997) *The social firms handbook,* Brighton: Pavilion Publishing.

Work experience and training

The project found that some people who wanted to get paid jobs were using 'day services' that had originally been set up as small businesses providing work experience and training for people with learning difficulties. The businesses, however, had not developed – and nor had any new opportunities for the people having work experience. Although people saw it as work they were not employees, were not being properly paid and were not gaining any qualifications to help their careers. The person-centred planning process highlighted that some residents were very dissatisfied with what they were doing in these services and wanted something different.

This is not an uncommon picture in small business projects that have been set up as a vehicle to provide work experience and training. The danger is that people move into such projects but fail to get the support they need to move on, either within the business or beyond it. There are some clear implications for people developing projects or placing people in them.

Commissioners need to:

- ensure that there are supported employment workers linked into work experience/training projects to help people move on to full employment

    or

- ensure that the business is planned and costed so that a work experience 'trainee' can move into a full 'employee' post within a reasonable period of time. This would mean most businesses having to support only a *very small* number of trainees if they are to both survive financially *and* employ people in meaningful roles central to the business

Care managers need to:

- ensure that people understand the nature of the placement and longer-term employment goals from the outset

    and

- monitor people in work experience/training placements to ensure that their experience and training is actually used to help them get a job. People in such placements require *active* care management

This is also an issue for many young disabled people who have gone from school to college but then not received support to secure work at the end of their course. Four young people living in the JRHT homes finished full-time college courses during the early days of the project. None received support to look for jobs before their courses ended. Local authorities could divert people from day services if they commissioned employment support linked into full-time college courses.

Work experience in ordinary work settings can also have its problems. At the start of the project three tenants were doing voluntary work set up as work experience placements, two in charity shops and one in a residential home for older people. Work experience may be appropriate where someone is unsure of the type of work they would like or wants to strengthen their curriculum vitae, but there are inherent dangers unless it is time-limited and linked to job-seeking support. For the three JRHT tenants their 'work experience' had been long-standing and there had been no discussion about next steps.

People are not receiving the support they need to get jobs because many providers of employment support take an approach that emphasises work 'readiness'. The problem is that many disabled people are never judged to be ready.

The growing number of supported employment schemes around the UK and America demonstrate that people do not need to be 'ready', they simply need the right support. Supported employment works. People requiring high levels of support can and do hold down paid jobs. The indications are that large numbers of disabled people who currently use day service provision would prefer to work. Ensuring that appropriate employment support is available is therefore a legitimate responsibility of local authorities.

Key action points for services

- Ensure senior managers give visible and vocal support for the idea of people having jobs

- Raise awareness among service users, staff in day and residential services *and* family carers that work is a viable option

- Build commitment by showing that supported employment is possible and does work for people with high support needs

- Refocus and redirect resources so that employment support is made available to people

- Ensure that when people say they want a job they get quick, face-to-face contact with an employment worker so that the moment is 'seized' and built on positively. This means having enough employment workers to meet the demand

- Give people clear, factual information about the effect of pay on a person's benefits

- Establish good working links with mainstream employment services and relevant funders

- Have an easy system within residential services for people to pay any shortfall in their 'rent' once they are receiving earnings from work instead of full benefits

What the project did

In the absence of a local supported employment agency the project employed its own employment workers. At the same time, however, it supported developments in the two local authorities so that supported employment provision would be strengthened.

The link between the person-centred planning process and employment support was crucial. It meant that people who were starting to talk to their planning circle about work could be responded to quickly and their interest nurtured and taken seriously.

Drawing on the local knowledge and contacts of staff across the residential homes greatly helped to identify potential work settings.

Investing in the training and support of the employment workers was important. Training in marketing skills paid off in the number and range of openings secured for people. Providing focused mentoring, separate from line management, from someone with substantial experience in supported employment ensured they received practice guidance as well as organisational direction.

Conrad writes:	Yvonne enjoyed going to the
I've got a job at a hotel in the kitchen. I work with Gavin and Joyce washing the dishes, putting them in the dishwasher and putting them away in the cupboards. I start at 7 pm and finish at 10 pm. I work on Wednesdays, Thursdays, Fridays, Saturdays and Sundays. I am really enjoying my job.	supermarket every Tuesday with her sister. She had got to know a few of the staff there. At her planning circle meeting she said she might like to work there. So, Yvonne tried out working in different areas of the supermarket to see which she liked. She decided she wanted to go for a paid job working with CDs and videos.

Becca gaining experience of work with older people

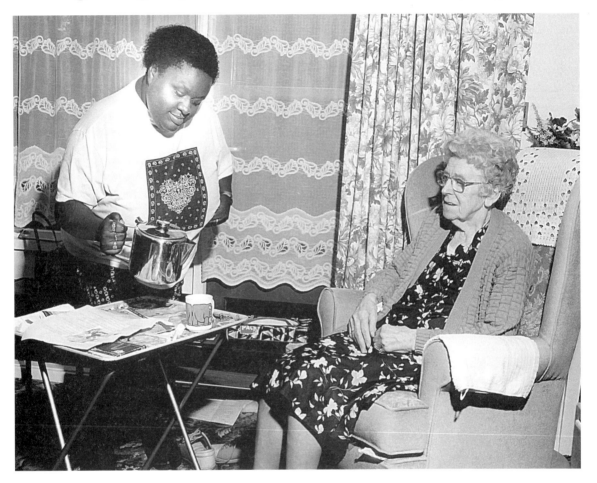

Job carving

One way that people achieve success in the workplace is by having a job that matches their particular talents and skills. Working with an employer to carve a job – to tailor-make it for an individual – is an important tool in supported employment. It can be seen as a 'reasonable adjustment' for an employer to make, under the provisions of the Disability Discrimination Act, in order to employ a disabled person. Job carving is about people getting real jobs, with a job description, contract and associated salary.

Job carving has implications for employers. There are two ways that it can be approached.

Option 1

New post created over and above existing posts, tailor-made for the disabled individual	The employer: • evaluates and puts a grade to the post (assigns a salary) • funds the post over and above existing posts

Option 2

New post created by splitting up (carving out) tasks from an existing post to tailor-make post for the disabled individual	The employer: • has, in effect, two new posts created from the previous one, so evaluates and puts grades to *both new posts* (assigns salaries) • funds the posts from the previously existing post

During the project it became clear that most employers:
- *are reluctant* to consider job carving once a job has already been advertised – they are simply keen to fill the post;
- *will* consider carving a job for someone if it's not paid or if the person wants to work for the £15 weekly earnings limit disregarded by the Benefits Agency.

This suggests that job carving should be:
- targeted towards employers who are known to be expanding or opening up a new business or branch; **or**
- part of an agreed plan with an established employer which aims to support a person from an unpaid work experience position into a paid job carved for them within a set period of time.

Job carving is about negotiating flexibility with employers – starting with duties and responsibilities that recognise a person's existing talents but building from there to support them to learn new tasks and expand their skills.

Job carving in action

The project worked closely with an employer to secure part-time paid employment for G through Option 2.

G loves being around books and paper and is skilled in spotting spelling mistakes and doing filing. He can also use a photocopier, computer and the telephone. He wanted to work in a fairly quiet environment in York, like an office or a library. The employer approached has a publications department and a library in their head office.

A clerical assistant's job description was used as the basis for the initial job carving. The duties and responsibilities of the post are shown below, with those that matched G's particular talents shown in bold and those that it was felt he could learn in italic.

1. Typing of standard letters, general correspondence and general secretarial support, audio and copy typing

2. **Answering the telephone**, *dealing with queries* and **sending out standard documents**

3. *Log claims onto system* and **match them with relevant files**

4. Secretarial support for X

5. *Support for the Director's PA*

6. **Responsibility for the Project filing system**

7. **Sorting, opening and distributing post for all staff**

8. *Being a key user for the photocopiers, maintaining their records* and **keeping them clean and stocked with paper**

9. Using the scanner to put proposals onto the word processing system

10. **Copying of standard documents and assisting with the production of Committee reports**

11. *Monitoring stocks of stationery, including stocking the printer daily*

12. *Other general tasks under the direction of the Director's PA*

There were no immediate vacancies so the employer agreed to a six-week period when G could 'taste' a range of departments in head office with a view to carving a job for him at the end of that period, ideally under Option 2 if a vacancy had arisen.

The national minimum wage

The introduction of a national minimum wage in April 1999 is being closely monitored to assess its impact on disabled people. A survey of Supported Employment agencies undertaken by AfSE on the first anniversary of the introduction of the minimum wage found that:

- 40% of disabled people who were working were still earning less than the minimum wage;

- the weekly pay of 19% of people had increased;

- increased earnings did not necessarily mean people were better off because they may have been losing benefits as a result;

- many people were no better off because they adjusted their working hours to compensate for the increased wage and keep their benefits;

- people were unhappy about reducing their hours;

- some agencies closed and people lost their jobs because of the minimum wage;

- some employers had taken no action to increase pay or were waiting for guidance.

Clearly the minimum wage has yet to be made to bite in terms of having a real impact on low paid disabled people.

Carol had been working in a voluntary capacity in a residential home for older people for several years, and was very keen to get paid for what she did. The project approached the manager who agreed to pay Carol, but only £15 for 12 hours. When the issue of the national minimum wage came up it was clear that it had not been considered in relation to Carol as a disabled person, and that the organisation would not implement it.

Benefits issues

At the time of writing disabled people continue to face a benefits trap when trying to move into employment. Many are effectively forced into pursuing the 'therapeutic earnings' route in order to safeguard other benefits and, even then, may see little if any extra cash in their pockets. The situation acts as a disincentive to people and creates very real anxiety.

The problems are outlined very clearly in the easy-to-read section of *Days of change:*

> Too often the person has to choose between having a job or having benefits. It is difficult to gradually reduce benefits as a person earns more in wages. If a person loses his/her job it can take a long time to get back on benefits.... We need to change the way benefits are organised so that disabled people can more easily take up job opportunities. (McIntosh and Whittaker, 1998)

When supporting people towards employment it is important to:

- Help each person get a *detailed* breakdown of the benefits they are receiving

- Look at each person's situation individually – don't assume that two people will be getting the same benefits

- Give the person information to help them understand the general benefits of working and any potential financial impact, and support them to make an informed decision about which way to proceed with earnings and benefits

- Give staff working with the person in residential and day services accurate information so that their anxieties about benefits are lessened too

- Give managers of residential services accurate information so that they can evaluate the potential impact on their fees income (revenue) and put systems or plans into place to address any shortfall

- Help people speak up to policy makers about the way they are disadvantaged by the system

Some of the issues faced by jobseekers from the homes highlighted the existing difficulties with national benefits policy. Most people were receiving Severe Disablement Allowance with an Income Support top up. Most were very fearful of losing their benefits and ending up worse off if they took up paid work. The project was acutely aware of the possibility that someone's eligibility for 'incapacity for work' benefits might be questioned if they were indeed doing some paid work. As Simons points out: "The benefit system is a minefield for people on incapacity benefits who want to explore the possibility of taking up paid work" (1998).

> For an overview of current problems and disincentives around benefits and work see: Simons, K. (1998) *Home, work and inclusion: The social policy implications of supported living and employment for people with learning disabilities*, York: Joseph Rowntree Foundation.

Supporting people to take part in more varied and ordinary leisure pursuits

Leisure is about relaxing, doing things we like doing, enjoying ourselves and having fun. It can be at home or away from home, on our own or with other people, gentle or active. It is a very personal choice and the leisure activities people want to pursue are incredibly wide-ranging.

Leisure pursuits also bring people together. A leisure activity is more than just the doing, it is also about sharing an interest with others and developing friendships and connections. Leisure pursuits can help prevent isolation and loneliness.

Key action points for services
Focus on integration and involvement

- Have objectives and outcome statements about leisure that stress integration and community involvement.

- Emphasise that supporting people to expand their leisure interests is not just about them doing an activity, but about doing it in ways and in places that will create a greater sense of belonging and connection with other people.

- Support people to do their chosen activity regularly – it is more likely to develop into a long-term interest and lead to new friendships.

- Support people to do things locally and in ordinary community settings so that there is an opportunity to build new friendships with people nearby.

- Deliberately create openings for people to talk about their leisure activities with others. Friendships often develop from sharing a common interest.

Does this mean we should stop people going to clubs or groups for disabled people?

No – but it is about redressing the balance and opening up other opportunities. In the past many people have *only* spent their leisure time with other disabled people. They were not offered other options. Deliberate action needs to be taken to ensure that people do things alongside other people in their local area too.

Ann has a very varied social life and contact with a lot of different people. She really enjoys going to an evening art class in the village every week with her friend Carol from the home and has met a lot of local people. She is also a member of the local Makaton choir and People First. Ann goes to church every Sunday. She has recently joined the Cliff Richard fan club and is hoping to see him in a concert soon.

Encourage new interests

- Disabled people have often had few opportunities to experience leisure activities outside their home. They therefore need information about a wide variety of leisure pursuits to 'broaden their horizons'. Hearing from other disabled people who have developed an active leisure life can be a valuable incentive. Staff also need to see that it is possible so that they will encourage the person in their choice of activities.

- New interests can be encouraged by giving people a chance to try new things. It means accepting that there may be false starts and changes of mind. It means recognising that people may dip in and out of things. For services this means staying alert to the quality of someone's leisure time. Person-centred planning really helps with this.

- Our leisure interests are often shaped by what is available near our home. For people who have difficulty reading or who don't get out and about in the community it is not easy to get information about local opportunities.

Ideas for getting information to people:

- Encourage them to watch TV programmes made by disabled people

- Use videos showing disabled people doing things

- Subscribe to newsletters and papers from organisations of disabled people

- Produce regular summary sheets of 'What's On' locally

- Subscribe to local newspapers

- Identify two users who can act as 'social secretaries' and support them to gather information from local libraries/shops/offices to share with everyone

- Set up a 'what's on' bulletin board

Create new opportunities

- All staff should be involved in looking for new leisure openings. They have a vast range of personal networks and connections that could be a way in to an activity for someone. It's a case of "I don't know anything about model car racing, but I know someone who does...". Getting staff teams to map and use their own connections can be a very positive way of increasing opportunities.

- However, it is also valuable to have someone whose job it is to find new opportunities. In York, the Leisure and Education Coordinator – a new post within day services – focuses on developing links with community groups and services to create more ordinary opportunities for people. Community Bridge Builders in other parts of the country have a similar role (see McIntosh and Whittaker, 1998, Chapter 6).

- Collating information from people's planning can show where targeted development is needed. An example of this occurred in York when a very high number of people said they wanted to go swimming regularly. This indicated that planned development was needed to make it happen. Evidence of unmet need is also helpful when applying for project funding through organisations like the Sports Council or the National Lottery.

- Leisure services are the responsibility of local councils. Disabled people and services supporting them can influence the development of such services by making their requirements known directly to corporate planners and politicians. Equality of opportunity is a key argument.

Provide flexible and reliable support

- Many ordinary leisure activities take place in the evenings and at weekends. Yet many disabled people only get to do them during the day. For example, people still attend discos during the day within day services – an activity more associated with children than adults. This type of thing continues to happen because services struggle to free up staff to provide support in the evenings and at weekends. This is an issue about the commissioning and purchasing of support for leisure activities.

Commissioning leisure services and support

Commissioners need to state clearly, in service specifications, their expectations on issues such as:

- Age-appropriate leisure activities taking place at age-appropriate times and in settings designed for those activities

- The role of day services in providing support vis-à-vis any residential providers and community support services locally

- The role of 'volunteers', unpaid supporters/buddies and 'natural supports' in people's leisure lives

- Providers actively seeking the other benefits that come from leisure activities such as friendships, learning and personal development, increased independence, relief for carers

---

- Whether or not enough support is available is also about how services are organised and the way staff are used. Few day or residential services have been set up to deliver support centred on what individuals want. To do so will require most services to reorganise so they can use their existing resources differently (see Chapter 8).
- Day, residential and community support services need to work together. Services can too easily get stuck in a 'passing the buck' culture where nothing gets done and nothing changes for the individual.

In York, the local day service agreed to take responsibility for supporting people in leisure activities they might want to do in their usual day service hours. If they wanted to do something in the evening or at weekends the residential service would support them.

In reality the day service found it difficult to free up staff during the day because they were supporting so many other people in groups. There was little flexibility because of the way the service was organised and staff were being used. A larger reorganisation was needed to achieve the flexibility required for individual activities.

Most of the improvements in people's leisure were achieved in the evenings and at weekends.

- Reliability and continuity of support is an important consideration. Most people had leisure interests from the past that they wanted to start again. Many had stopped purely because the member of staff supporting them had left. Person-centred planning can help with monitoring and rectifying this situation if necessary. However, it is no substitute for the service organisation carefully planning staff work tasks around people's individual goals.

Deliberately nurture relationships

- It is important to think beyond paid staff in building connections for people in the community. Providing support does not have to be about employing more staff (see Chapter 7 for further discussion of this point).

Address the cost of leisure activities

- Increased leisure activities almost inevitably bring increased costs – membership fees, equipment/materials, travelling expenses, refreshments. People need information about the costs so that they can make choices about how they spend their money.

- Services should ensure that people are supposed to maximise their income, particularly through benefit checks.

- A number of financial breaks are available to disabled people that can make the cost of leisure easier to bear, like reduced-price leisure cards, bus passes, railcards; again, information for staff is important so that they can support people to apply.

- Managing charitable offers, such as free block tickets for the theatre, can be a dilemma. Talk directly to the person making the offer and try to negotiate a compromise that is more focused on individuals.

- Try negotiating with leisure and transport providers for reduced charges in the form of 'companion passes' for supporters.

Supporting people to learn more and increase their independence

Learning can take place anywhere, at any time and at any age. The project found that age was certainly no barrier to people's desire to learn. Opportunities, however, are shaped by services and there are continuing issues around choice, support and the culture for learning.

Formal educational opportunities and support

The term formal educational opportunities is used here to mean those provided through adult education classes and further/higher education courses. These are still difficult for many disabled people to make use of because:

- courses emphasise achievement and progression based on traditional assessment methods and standard completion times; many disabled people need to be able to show their learning in different ways, in smaller steps and over a longer period of time;

- individualised support is hard to secure – colleges receive funding for support that is based on the assessed needs of students, but most use it to employ general class assistants rather than targeting it to individuals; day and residential services find it difficult to provide support staff to accompany people to classes.

The result is that people needing higher levels of support because of their degree of disability are effectively excluded.

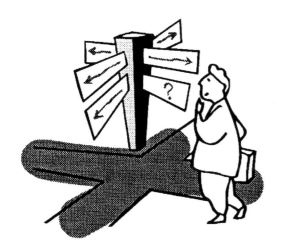

For people with learning disabilities there can be additional problems about college provision targeted specially for them:

- what is available is not necessarily linked to information about what people want – the same options are offered year-on-year;
- because there is 'special' provision most people do not get to know about the full range of classes available; they tend to get filtered towards the special provision and the enormously diverse range of adult education provision, in particular, is not considered.

Improved collaboration between education and 'care' providers is needed at three levels:

Senior level: Senior managers need to develop a shared strategic direction, particularly around inclusion, and agree resource allocation. It is important that senior managers within care agencies understand the decision-making and management structure of their local education provider(s) so that they can make links at the appropriate level to achieve change.

> Agree inclusion strategy, and resources to support it

Operational management level: In many areas there is a culture of blame that gets in the way of joint problem solving, not helped by relatively infrequent contact between education and care staff. People need to meet regularly to focus on areas of joint concern and work together more effectively. For example, link up information from the separate individual planning systems used and devise innovative assessment approaches together.

> Link up individual planning systems, agree new learning assessment methods and bring staff together

Service delivery level: Work with education colleagues to make something happen for one person at a time. Make personal links with tutors and get them involved in people's individual planning.

> Work together to make something different happen for one person at a time

> Jonathan's tutor from the local agricultural college joined his planning circle. He was going to a course one day a week but it became clear that he wanted more. This led to him joining another course and also getting weekend work experience on a farm.

Information for users and staff on the full range of course/class opportunities

Unless staff get information they can't support people to look at it and consider their options. It is rare that all the information about courses and classes in a locality is found together because there may be several different organisations running them. It helps to have someone who can seek out all the information, put it into an accessible format and then distribute it. The range of distance learning opportunities should also be included: some people may prefer to do their learning at home.

Leadership and direction

Staff in care services need continuous encouragement to look beyond special provision and consider educational options that are open to all members of the public. They need to know that this is expected. Tutors and relatives need to understand this too. Managers must be prepared to help resolve any practical difficulties. Positive leadership is sometimes about showing people that there *is* a way through.

> Geoffrey enjoys history and wanted to go to an evening class to learn more about antiques. He enrolled in a local class and was supported to attend the first few sessions. Some people were anxious that Geoffrey might have difficulties in a class open to members of the public – but he soon dispelled any worries. Geoffrey's knowledge of history means he can contribute actively to the class and he is welcomed as a member of the group.

Dennis at his weekly Internet class

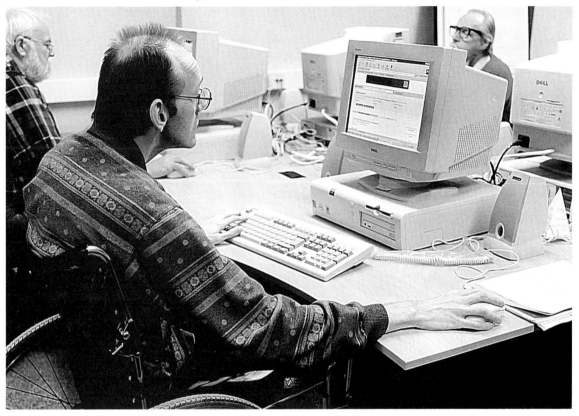

Planning creatively to provide learning support

The planning comes in working out what support a person might need in a class, targeting support towards those areas and then regularly reviewing the support needed. As people get used to a setting and the people around them they often need less support. The creativity comes in thinking about all the different ways that someone could get the support they need.

Here are some possibilities:

- People training as volunteers (as part of their course)

- People training as teachers, social workers and so on

- Staff from day or residential services

- A support worker specifically recruited for the task

- Other class students acting as 'buddies'

- A friend who goes with the person to the class

Some of these options cost money – which may mean using existing resources differently. Some of the options are about building informal supports. Some are about partnerships.

The service culture

People often talk about organisations having a 'learning culture'. The emphasis should be on supporting staff to reflect on and learn from what they do, try out new ideas and give and receive feedback. Supporting disabled people to learn more and increase their independence is also about services having a learning culture – one where every moment spent supporting a person is viewed as a potential opportunity for the person to learn and develop. The following strategies can help to build such a culture.

Taking deliberate action to create the culture

This must be planned action to achieve change – and it has to be about everyone. Staff will not respond positively if they are expected to support people to learn but don't feel that they themselves are being supported to learn and develop or if they are regularly facing organisational obstacles. A learning culture requires a focus on enabling rather than 'caring for', attention to risk management and leaders who have a developmental approach (see Chapter 3).

Supporting staff to acquire the skills to help people learn

It is often assumed that staff instinctively know how to help people learn. This is wrong because there are specific techniques that assist with learning and people do not automatically use them. It can also be dangerous because if someone doesn't seem to be learning it might be assumed they are not able to, rather than that the approach is not right for them.

Every moment spent with a person presents a learning opportunity but staff need to know how to turn the opportunity into a learning experience. One way of ensuring that staff have some knowledge is to incorporate specific training into the service induction process.

When the project organised a one-day workshop on 'Helping people learn' staff felt it really helped them understand what they needed to do. They felt they should have had the information much earlier in their careers.

"Everyone should get this input. We all needed it at the start of our jobs."

Two important areas for staff training are systematic instruction techniques and how to assess and manage risks.

Systematic instruction

Systematic instruction involves breaking tasks down into steps and methodically supporting people to learn them. It is regularly used by supported employment workers to help people learn specific work tasks but is a useful approach in any learning situation.

For more information contact:
TSI (Training in Systematic Instruction) Ltd
Ashleigh
Sunnyside
Todmorden
Lancashire
OL14 7AP

Training on how to assess and manage risks
Training is likely to be most effective if it:

- is linked to, and reinforces a clear policy and risk management process;

- is given to managers first, and then involves them in training their staff;

- helps people understand *why* it's important and how everyone can gain;

- tutors people through some examples based on their own experience with individuals;

- incorporates follow-up to develop people's actual practice and help them do it well.

Formal training helps staff develop their knowledge but development of skills needs to be practice-based. It is the interplay of knowledge and skills that leads to competent practice. On-the-job supervision, reflection and feedback is essential.

Organising staff time around the goals and aspirations of individuals
A common complaint from staff is that they don't have much time to focus on supporting individuals. This is often a reflection of the way their time is organised. Person-centred planning spotlights this issue.

The project found that the introduction of person-centred planning, with its very individualised focus, signalled the need for staff to be deployed differently – both in the residential and the day services. Initially, both services and staff felt under pressure until different ways of using staff began to be introduced.

To help people learn staff need to be actively engaged with them. This means being focused on the person and the task or situation that they are facing. It means continually asking the question 'What is the person getting out of this?'. Being actively engaged is about empowering people. It is not about staff having a list of tasks that have to be done, and simply getting through them. One tool that has been shown to help with organising and focusing staff time around goals and outcomes for people is Active Support.

Active Support is

... about recognising that every moment has potential, and supporting people to undertake real, everyday activities at home and in the community. It is about enabling people to do things themselves ... actively engaging people in daily activities. It requires teamwork, especially regular team planning of staff time to ensure that people are supported to do things and achieve their goals. (Pavilion Publishing, 1987; Felce, 1996).

Many day and residential services employ ancillary staff to prepare meals, clean and look after the buildings, do grounds maintenance, and so on. Person-centred planning in York showed that many people using services want to develop their own skills in these areas. Services need to review their use of ancillary staff so they open up more learning opportunities for people and a chance to develop greater independence.

Supporting people to have greater control over their life

If you learn how to do something yourself you ultimately have more control over it. But having more control is not just about doing things, it is also about making decisions.

In York people wanted to do things for themselves such as:
- Cooking
- Using the buses
- Shopping
- Using the telephone
- Tying their shoelaces
- Wording letters
- Going to the library to choose a talking book

People wanted to start making their own decisions about:
- Where to have their hair done
- Where to go on holiday, and who with
- What they do and how often they go to day services
- Where to live in the future

In the person-centred planning process we found that it was some time before people started identifying things they wanted more control over. When you are used to receiving services that are familiar and smooth running, it can be difficult to contemplate major lifestyle changes. The planning circles needed encouragement to help people think in terms of activities and decisions that would really put them more in charge of their lives. Staff and people involved in planning with individuals need to think 'beyond the comfort zone' if people are to gain more control over their lives.

They need to be challenged to think about:
- Who does what for the person
- What more the person could be supported to do
- Who decides what for the person
- What decisions the person could take charge of or be more involved in

Leaders and managers need to think about:
- What might be preventing people taking more control
- How the service can be changed to enable this to happen

Everyday choices	Lifestyle decisions
What shall I wear? What do I want to eat? Do I want a hot or a cold drink? Shall I watch the TV or listen to music? Shall I have a beer or a fruit juice? Shall I go to bed now or a bit later?	Do I want to look after my own money? Do I want to use public transport to get around? Do I want to try to get a job? Do I want to move into different accommodation? Do I want to live with my boyfriend? Do I want to be vegetarian?

Services that successfully support people to take as much control as they can over their life do many of the following:

- **Ensure people get information** in accessible formats so that they are aware of the range of lifestyle choices and can make informed decisions

- **Support and promote self-advocacy** and speaking up forums

- **Train and develop their staff** to support and interact with someone in an empowering way

- **Focus on people's rights** as citizens, and associated responsibilities

- **Provide clear direction, leadership and active management** that reinforces the goal to staff and supports them putting it into practice

- **Introduce easier systems** so that people can do more for themselves

- **Provide, create or adapt aids** so that people can do more for themselves and/or communicate more easily

- Give attention to how they can **help people learn new skills**

- **Actively manage risks**

- **Develop a total culture of empowerment** so they give *consistent* messages to users about being in control of their life

- **Create opportunities** for people to be in control, for example involving people in recruitment of staff, developing peer support networks

- **Devolve finances** to people so they have real power and control

Control of personal finances

Imagine not having money in your pocket and having to ask someone else every time you want to buy anything. Certainly difficult for the average person to contemplate – but this is still the reality for many disabled people. It is not just that people are poor because of living on benefits. It is also about who controls the money they do have. People get a greater sense of having control over their own life if they are handling their own money.

There is a lot of fear about people handling their own money:

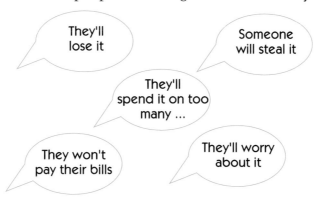

The fear can be dealt with by paying attention to risk management and helping people learn. Services can put systems and processes into place that support people to handle their own money safely. What is needed is a fundamental commitment to empowering people and a determination to work through the operational issues and problems that arise.

It is equally important that people who need significant levels of support are seen to be in charge of their own money. Even the fact of them carrying it themselves gives a clear message that it is *the person's* money, and helps to reinforce that they are the customer and therefore a person to be treated with respect.

Control and people with complex needs

Helping people with more complex needs and communication difficulties to have greater control over their life is a significant challenge for services. Supporting someone to do as much as possible for him/herself is an important starting point.

- Aids and adaptations that are tailored to the individual can make an enormous difference to the level of control they have.

- Staff having a detailed understanding of how someone communicates is fundamental to recognising their own choices and decisions.

Decisions do have to be made on behalf of some individuals. Many services support people where their capacity to make decisions is (or becomes) an issue, and yet they do not directly address this in their framework documents. It is left unclear how they will deal with decision making – who will be involved and in what kind of decisions. This is an area that many services could usefully clarify.

People who have deteriorating health may be particularly at risk of having major lifestyle decisions made for them. When someone is ill the desire to care for and protect them becomes more pronounced. The temptation to make decisions *away* from the person can be strong, for genuinely caring reasons. This may be reinforced by the behaviour of medical practitioners who talk to the carers rather than the person.

The role of circles in decision making

Where people have the backing of a planning circle or a circle of support there is a ready-made group of people with the person's interests at heart who can be involved in decision making. This is particularly helpful for people with complex needs.

A shared approach to decision making can help to ensure that everyone's views are heard without dominating those of the central person. It helps services have a clear rationale and the authority to take action on behalf of individuals. It helps relatives to feel involved in decision making. For residential services it can lead to a more effective partnership with relatives. The project found that most people wanted their relatives to be involved in major decisions about their lives and that person-centred planning circles were an effective way of achieving this.

Service design

The design of a service can have a major impact on the extent to which people can exercise control over their own lives. This is an important issue for commissioners, which is examined in more detail in Chapter 8.

Redesigning an existing service can be a daunting task, but it may be necessary in order to create opportunities for people to have more control over their lives. Residential services not based on domestic-sized accommodation, and day services supporting large numbers of people together, create dilemmas about individual control in relation to the wishes of the larger group. The smaller the number of people doing things together the easier it is to manage such issues.

7

Building relationships through community involvement

Successfully including people in their local community and seeing them develop a network of friends and neighbourhood connections was one of the major themes underlying all the Changing Days work. Most service policy documents state that they have this aim for the people they serve, but in practice organisations seem to find this difficult to achieve and many disabled people still lead relatively segregated and limited social lives. As *Changing days* puts it:

> A vision of inclusiveness will demand major shifts in the way we think and act – as individuals, in organisations and as members of our local communities. (Wertheimer, 1996)

What is 'community'?

When people talk about 'my community' they may be thinking of very different things. It might be a geographical area either close to where they live or, in this age of travel and communication technology, it can stretch to being world-wide. There are many 'communities of interest' within which people share an interest in work, leisure, learning or commitment to particular causes or groups. There are communities which share a common culture or life experience, sometimes centred around ethnicity or age. Community is not just a place, but a set of connections or ties we have with other people. Having ties and connections to others is important to the vast majority of people. *Ties and connections* (King's Fund, 1988) set out the following list of important sources of ties and connections:

- Friendship
- Acquaintance
- Membership
- Keeping in touch
- Being part of a family
- Having a partner
- Being a neighbour
- Knowing or being known in a neighbourhood

Some of these 'ties and connections' are strong and mean a great deal to us, others are weaker but form a significant part of the ebb and flow of our lives. All are important in building a sense of who we are and where we belong. Many disabled people have never had the chance to develop strong ties other than family ties and even those may have been broken very early in their lives. They are also likely to have experienced more than the average number of changes and disruptions in their lives, many of which will have meant loss of 'connections' with other people. They may have lost contact with friends through being moved from institution to institution, or when they have moved from an institution to a new home in the community. They lose contact with staff as people move on to other jobs. The challenge is to get people out of the 'service-centred' life, largely governed by the needs of the organisation, to a more person-centred, community-based life. Doing so means that they have more control and can expect to have more continuity and depth to their relationships.

The situation in York

It was a distinct advantage to be working with people directly from their homes. They were already 'in the community' and many had close ties with their families. However, many still led fairly segregated lives, using special services for disabled people and having most of their 'ties and connections' with people they lived with, and with staff in the homes and the day services.

What helped?

The person-centred planning process did much to link people up with other local citizens, make new connections and re-connect with past people and interests. The planning circles helped to bring people together, particularly from the local community.

Many of the advantages are set out in detail in other chapters (see particularly the section on Leisure in Chapter 6, pages 69-74).

There are a number of other ways of working which can help to strengthen people's ties and connections in all their variety.

Be persistent and focus on talents

Making connections for people can take time. It is important not to give up and to be willing to try again or try a different way when a breakthrough to an opportunity does not happen first time around.

How the initial approach is made can make the difference between success and failure. For example, emphasising to a community group or organisation that the person has talents to offer and can contribute.

> Ian grew up in a family where acting and the theatre were important and valued. Both his parents are professional actors. Ian has inherited this interest and has appeared on screen as a paid extra in a number of productions, including Emmerdale. What Ian most wanted to do was join a local drama group and be involved in productions more regularly, so people in Ian's planning circle enthusiastically approached some local drama groups. Initially the responses were very disappointing. It did not seem that any group would welcome Ian and people were close to giving up.
>
> The breakthrough came when people changed what they were saying when approaching a group. Instead of asking them to help Ian, they focused on Ian being able to help the drama group – the talents he had to offer. He has now been written into the script of the drama group's next production and is rehearsing two evenings a week. He is over the moon and making new contacts in his local community.

It may take a lot of 'leg work' before success is achieved.

> One of the person-centred planning facilitators visited 10 different charity shops to talk to them about voluntary work for Ann. She came up with four possibilities. Ann then visited them and made her choice.

Ann at the till in the Fairer World shop

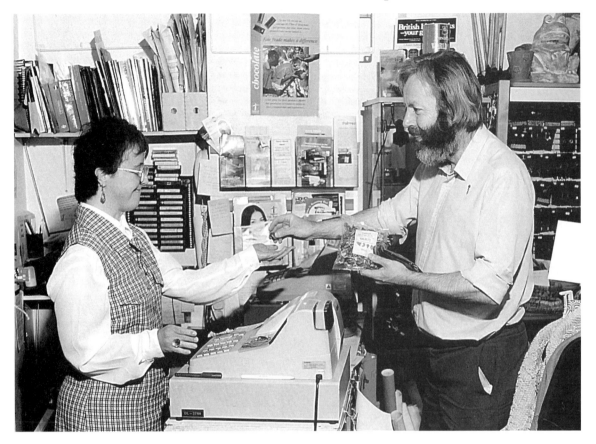

Do not be afraid to ask

Helping someone make contact with new people in the community can be simply about asking. Start with the assumption that there is someone out there who will be willing, and it's just a matter of tracking that person down. It happened for Andrew....

> Andrew likes animals of all kinds and sizes. He told his planning circle that he really wanted to look after a dog. It's not easy to own a dog when you live with 12 other people, so two people from his circle went out in search of someone with a dog that Andrew could get to know. They asked local dog owners and soon found a man who was happy for Andrew to join him in walking his dog one evening a week. Andrew, dog and owner are getting on fine.

Plan well and be prepared for the unexpected

Helping to achieve someone's goal is easier if there is good planning and preparation. It is important to try and be prepared for the unexpected. It helps to think through how the person may be affected if something goes wrong and have some alternative strategies to draw on.

> Joyce wanted to have her hair done regularly at a local hairdressing salon. Members of her planning circle helped her arrange a hairdressing appointment in a salon in the town, and at the appointed time she and a member of staff set off. The staff member on this occasion was a relief worker who only knew that Joyce had an appointment that she had made herself. When they got into town it became clear that Joyce couldn't remember the name of the salon. Undaunted, the worker went with Joyce from salon to salon until they found the right one. Joyce achieved her goal, and has gone on to make regular appointments there.

In contrast...

> John wanted to improve his literacy skills and went with a worker into the nearby town to enquire about a course run by a particular organisation. When they arrived they found that the organisation was not at the address they had, so they turned round and went home again. Luckily John did not give up so easily. He rang the organisation, found their new address and enrolled himself on his chosen course.

Give people valued roles

An important part of being included is actively participating in an event or activity. It is about being given the opportunity to 'give' as well as 'take'. Using our gifts and skills in a way which is helpful to others increases our own enjoyment and satisfaction. Having a job to do can be a good way of 'breaking the ice' in new situations with new people.

> Toby was already going to church but wanted to be more involved. The vicar, who was a member of his circle, suggested that he might like to help give out the hymn books before the service. This has led to Toby becoming much more involved in other activities of the church, including the youth groups.

Eileen in her role as Assistant with the Brownies

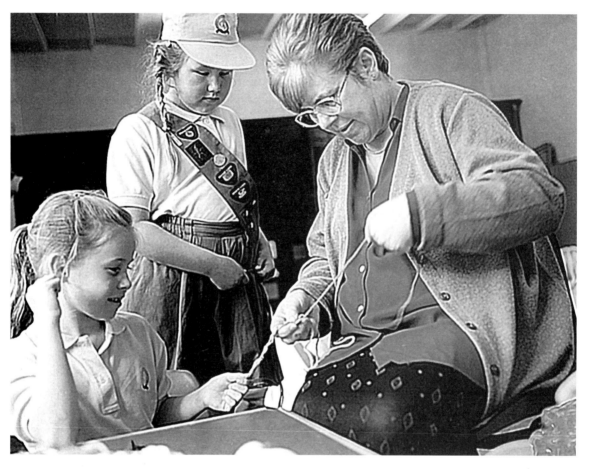

Explore all the options

Sometimes it will be necessary to do some detective work to uncover all the options which might lead to achieving a person's goal. This involves going further than just investigating the first thing that springs to mind.

> Mary wanted to go to see films regularly. People supporting her knew about one club, but it was specifically for disabled people. They decided to search further. They found out about the local cinemas and also some other film clubs – and were then able to give Mary the widest possible choice.

Deliberately nurture relationships

It is important to think beyond paid staff in building connections for people in the community. Supporting someone to be involved in a group or activity does not have to be about employing more staff. Pressure on resources would make this difficult to achieve anyway. We need to always be seeking to build natural supports – support from people who are not paid to be with the person. It could be someone who uses the same gym or stables, or someone who wants to share an allotment, for example.

Staff and members of planning circles may need a lot of encouragement to think about these wider connections. Staff are so used to the support patterns of services, they can find it difficult to think creatively about involving non-service people. Worries about risk and who carries the responsibility need to be addressed appropriately. The support of managers is crucial in 'giving permission' for this to happen. Planning circle members may be worried that they will be imposing on their friends and acquaintances. But it doesn't have to be about expecting other people to give a lot of time. It can be just about using their knowledge and connections to open doors to new opportunities for individuals.

Friendships and further contacts can result from these connections, thus widening and deepening people's ordinary links with the community.

Carol has made some good friends through her involvement in a home for older people

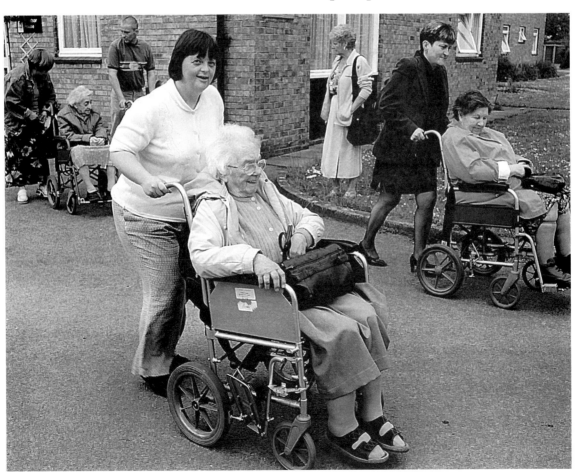

Conclusion

We cannot expect to achieve major changes in people's community connections overnight but we are learning much more about how to work differently in order to give people the maximum chance to be accepted and valued as other citizens. We cannot change society overnight so that every person is willing to welcome and include disabled people, but we do know that there are people in every community willing to be involved and, given time, persistence and mutual support, we can find them.

8
Changing services and support

"Change … is only another word for growth, another synonym for learning. We can all do it, and enjoy it, if we want to."
Charles Handy, 1989

Improving lives

To respond to what disabled people are saying they want in their lives means looking at how they will get support they need. It means examining whether existing services are set up in the best way to provide that support.

Four key actions are required of commissioners and service providers:
- Reorganise resources to achieve more flexible support

- Focus resources on individuals

- Create more ordinary community opportunities and natural supports for people

- Ensure organisations work collaboratively and creatively together

Person-centred planning works!

After 18 months the project found that there had been a significant change in the daily pattern of life for some people. This change meant that services were being used differently.

- More people were being supported to do things at or from home during the week. Some people said they really wanted to be at home for a day rather than out all week. Some wanted to do other things with their time. Some were waiting for work or college opportunities to be arranged.

Changes

At the start		After 18 months	
Number of days people were supported from home Monday to Friday	Number of people	Number of days people were supported from home Monday to Friday	Number of people
None	21	None	12
One	10	One	15
Two	6	Two	7
Three	4	Three	5
Four	1	Four	2
Five	0	Five	1

This change had implications for JRHT. Some staff were already on duty in the homes during the day but to provide more support meant changing the way the Trust used their overall staffing hours.

The number of people using, both local authority and independent sector day services, decreased, because people had chosen to pursue other opportunities. The changes were mainly in the York area.

At the start of the project 25 residents were using day services provided and/or purchased by City of York Community Services. 18 months later:

- 24 people were using day services provided and/or purchased by City of York Community Services

- 15 people had changed their day service use in some way – nine had reduced their use, four were using services for the same number of days but differently, and two had increased their use by one day a week

- Of the 15, two people had completely *moved out* of day services, offset by one person who had *started* using a service one day a week

What this meant for day services

17 days of service per week had been freed up, the equivalent of 3.4 full-time places across all the day services. This broke down to 10 days of service freed up within the in-house day service, and seven days of service freed up within independent sector contracted services.

Resource issues

Through the person-centred planning people had chosen a variety of different daytime activities – work, volunteering, going to college, sometimes staying at home. Some people needed only a small amount of ongoing support. The investment of time and energy largely focused on setting up new opportunities and supporting people to settle in. Most support was provided by JRHT and project staff, with some input from the local authority Community Link project.

The short-term investment in increased support paid off in longer-term gains for individuals and in freeing up places in day services for other people needing a service.

Based on a (low) hypothetical unit cost of £25 per day for a day service place (£6,325 per annum per full-time place) the freeing up of 3.4 places can be translated into a gross financial saving to the local authority of £21,505 (the unit cost of a place in a local authority social education/day centre for people with learning difficulties was calculated as £39 per day for 1996/97; Netten and Dennett, 1997). Logically this should show as savings in the care management purchasing budget. People needing day services can take up the vacancies created, thus achieving a saving against funds earmarked for new day service support packages. However, the picture is rather more complicated. Several key factors have to be taken into account.

- People moving away from established day services tend to be those needing lower levels of support, but those referred in recent years tend to need higher levels of support. This means that 'vacancies' may present an opportunity for provider services to renegotiate their staff-to-user ratios with commissioners so that they can give people better support. This happened in York. In such situations the agreed number of users to be supported by the service often decreases – the vacancies disappear. The danger is that these services then become 'special needs units' by accident.

- A community care assessment based on a person-centred lifestyles approach leads to a more specific picture of the opportunities and support a person wants and needs. The older established day services may not be organised to meet those requirements. Care managers may therefore choose not to purchase support from services if they cannot respond to what people want and need.

- The person-centred planning process, and the whole approach to support that goes alongside it, requires committed resources. It is an up-front investment that takes time before it reaps benefits for people, and for services. As an estimate, to introduce and support a person-centred planning process for 30 people would require funding in the first year to cover:

- a full-time planning facilitator
- management costs
- training
- expenses.

Add to this the need to free staff up from existing duties to become active participants in people's planning circles, and any costs associated with supporting people to achieve their goals.

- Supporting people with more complex needs to access a greater range of opportunities is likely to cost more and be needed longer. It is easier to achieve change for people needing lower levels of support because the support organisations do not have to change very much. Organisations will need to change more to be able to provide the necessary support for people with more complex needs. The lesson is that changes in people's lives will be limited by the extent to which organisations are willing to change themselves.

Reorganising day services

The way services are designed and organised has a fundamental impact on the opportunities and support open to a person. Experience indicates that better lifestyles for people are likely to be achieved if:

- *The service stays small:* The more people supported by a service the more difficult it is to stay focused on individuals.

- *It does not use large 'special' buildings:* The more buildings are owned and used by the service, the more finance is taken up in maintaining those buildings; also, large buildings used only by service users are more likely to cut people off from the local community.

- *It has autonomy:* The larger and more complex the agency the more likely it is that services will get distracted from their purpose by wider organisational management issues and slow down decision making.

But how can these things be achieved when the starting point is a provider service that supports well over a hundred people in two or three large buildings – centres or workshops – still a very common scenario around the UK today?

Days of change highlights the steps that can help to make this possible.

Days of change:

Step-by-step from day centres to community

Raise awareness; what's good about the day service?
What needs to change?

Get agreement from senior managers, elected members,
board members for changes.

Set up a 'change' group to steer the way forward.
Involve users, community members, employers, staff and carers.
Develop a communication strategy which keeps people
informed about and involved with changes.

Staff development to move a person-centred service which supports
individuals to participate in ordinary activities in an inclusive community.
Undertake person-centred plans (PCPs).
Develop circles of support for each person.

Hold a stakeholders' conference to engage a wide group of people
in the change process and capture their ideas for the future.
Visit examples of innovation and good practice.

Use outcomes from person-centred plans and information from
stakeholders' conferences to draft a framework for future services.
Create new job descriptions for staff.

Move resources (staffing and finance) to individual support for users
(direct payments), invest in supported employment and
community-based opportunities.

Get started helping people (one-by-one) to participate in new
activities, jobs and education opportunities.
Ensure risk assessments are used to minimise problems.

Find new alliances for additional funding
(eg TEC, Welfare to Work programmes, corporate sponsorship).

Measure improvement in people's lives by looking at original PCPs.
Improve opportunities.

Support – the core issue

Helping people lead more fulfilling lives means ensuring they get the support they need to achieve their personal goals. This requires more support than is currently available in most services and family support networks and is one of the major hurdles to overcome to achieve change. Unless additional core funding can be drawn into the service the main way that extra support can be funded is by using existing resources in different ways.

Ways to increase the amount of support available

- Apply for funding for employment support for individuals and projects from regeneration schemes, European funds and mainstream employment grants such as Access to Work

- Free up money used to pay for the upkeep and running of buildings

- Ensure that staff time is focused on contact with people using the service – not on paperwork and bureaucracy!

- Make links with staff in community facilities like leisure centres, youth clubs and libraries. Draw them into giving support to their 'customers'

- Provide student placements and offer student projects – not just to people on care, social work or nursing courses. Consider people on community work courses and students studying drama, art, sport, computing and other subjects disabled people might be interested in

- Train and support staff to build people's community networks and to foster natural supports

- Change job descriptions to create roles that are more person-centred and that have varying levels of responsibility. Create trainee or apprentice posts with a career structure that will attract people into the work

- Work creatively with providers of education and leisure services: pool resources to develop support so that people can take advantage of the opportunities they offer

- Think of focused projects that fall within national or local priorities and apply for funding from any source possible – throw as many balls in the air as possible!

Tackling the major changes

"It's about moving the titanic around"
(Local Authority Manager)

The two steps that involve the most organisational change are disinvesting from service buildings and changing the roles and responsibilities of staff. These can appear daunting, particularly as they may generate resistance from people who use and work in the service. However, unless they are tackled, the service's ability to provide more flexible and individual support will be limited.

Freeing up resources for more support by disinvesting from existing day centre buildings needs:

- positive and committed leadership
- good planning
- active management.

It is important to:

- Help people who use the service and their carers to think and dream about how the person's life could be improved and the support they would need for this to happen
- Be open about what the service would need to do to provide the necessary support
- Have managers and leaders who have a relationship with service users and their carers and take time to talk to them about service developments
- Enable people to take an active part in contributing to possible options for service change – consultation on its own is not enough
- Be clear that the nature of large group services means that change involves a certain amount of compromise if the services are to respond more to what individuals want
- Ensure that the impact of change is monitored, and that there are mechanisms in place to rapidly address any issues that arise

What should a reorganised service look like?

There is no simple answer! The reorganisation and redesign of any service will be based on local factors – the opportunities people want and the support they need, commissioning and purchasing priorities, other provision in the locality and the nature of the local community.

However, there seem to be some common features of successful person-centred services in the UK and the US:

- Staff are organised and focused on individuals or small numbers of people
- There is a teamwork approach. Decision making takes place at team level in partnership with service recipients and budgets are managed at team level
- Service leaders are close to, and engaged with service delivery
- The service develops partnerships with others. There is an outward-looking, innovative, action-learning culture

Changing residential services

Recent research into the quality and costs of residential supports for people with learning difficulties (Emerson et al, 1999) found that "smaller and more homely settings were associated with greater choice, greater access to leisure and community activities ... and reduced risk of abuse". *Facing the facts* (DoH, 1999) recommended national objectives for health and social care services, with medium-term targets to include "a reduction in the overall proportion of supported residents living in accommodation which is not of domestic scale or character". There is a growing national impetus for residential services to change the character of their provision.

The project was operating within a residential service. The four homes were not of a domestic scale but they were still people's homes – and many people were keen to say in their planning circle meetings that they liked living there. This is no great surprise: moving home is a big event for any of us, and it can be one of the most stressful life changes. Most of us need a good reason to consider moving home – a job change, we need more space, we want to be nearer family or friends. But such options are rarely discussed with people in residential homes. Once placed in a residential home, most people remain there for life.

Residential service providers can improve people's lives by changing the services they run, but this has implications for people living in their existing homes. Simply closing a home on a set date and moving everyone into smaller houses is unlikely to be very person-centred. Some people will be excited about moving and keen to do it, others will not. They and their relatives may feel unsure or frightened, and some will simply not want to consider other options. Also, people will want to live in different types of accommodation. Some will choose to live on their own and some with other people.

Changing a residential service in a way that is right for the people who live in the homes means:

- **Giving people information** about alternative ways of living and listening to what they want for themselves through a person-centred planning process.

- **Taking account of people's friendships and bonds,** and the tensions in relationships.

- **Managers and staff being positive about people moving on** so that people are encouraged to explore other options and express their preferences.

- **Using people's individual preferences** to shape the development of alternative forms of supported accommodation while continuing to run existing homes.

- **Helping people move on from a home gradually** rather than all at once.

- **Making a decision to stop accommodating new people** in homes when vacancies arise.

- **Planning for, and actively managing the funding issues** that arise because of the need to support people still in the homes as others move out.

- **Managing the use and security of the building** as the numbers of people reduce and areas are no longer used.

- **Ensuring that relationships and bonds between residents and staff are recognised** and built on when planning support for people.

One of the most difficult situations is where several people decide to move out leaving a small number who do not want to move on or whose families do not want them to. It is likely that some people will change their minds as they see where former residents are living and what their lives are like, but others may not. This leaves some people living in far from ideal conditions, in a building that is far too large and which has rooms or whole areas unused. There will also be budgetary implications for the organisation and issues that arise in relation to registration and inspection of the home.

One option may be to turn part of the building into a self-contained flat (or flats) for the remaining people, and demolish the remainder or use it differently. The disruption to people's lives by building works could potentially be managed by people taking holidays at key times during the works and with clear contracting and planning with the builders. It could present an opportunity for people to be very involved in the creation of their new home.

The fundamental requirement is that people have the opportunity to talk through the options, supported by (or, in the case of people with complex needs, represented by) people who care about them.

Person-centred planning constantly reminds us that each person is an individual with his/her own preferences and dreams and this needs to be recognised, even in congregate residential settings. It is not unusual to hear staff and relatives say "*people* don't want to move", "*everyone's* happy here", "*they* would be unsafe". Person-centred planning challenges those statements by hearing and valuing what each individual wants and finding ways to achieve their goals.

From residential service to supported living

Andy lives in a residential home with eight other disabled people but would now like to move on. He wants to live with someone, preferably a man near his own age, but doesn't have a really close friend in the home that he would want to share with. He wants some support – he feels a bit anxious about moving out of the home where there are staff to call on day and night. He doesn't want staff around all the time, just to help with particular things and to be 'on call' in case of emergencies.

Andy likes the area he lives in and wants to stay there. He also wants to be able to keep in touch with the people in the home. He wants a ground floor flat or one that has a lift so that he will be able to move around easily.

Helping Andy to get what he wants is what the concept of supported living is all about (Kinsella, 1993) It is a person-centred approach based on finding out how people want to live, identifying the support they need to live in that way, and then making it happen. It's about helping people to become tenants or owners of a property, with associated rights – and the control of their own home that goes with those rights. It is *not* about deciding to develop a number of supported group homes and then moving people into them because it's the only option they are given.

Supported Living emphasises:

- Separating out housing provision from support provision
- Focusing on one person at a time
- Full user choice and control
- Including everyone, rejecting no one
- The importance of community connections and natural supports

The Mental Health Foundation Committee of Enquiry into Services and Opportunities for people with learning difficulties welcomed developments in supported living:

> Housing arrangements should be tailored to individual need. Arrangements should be found for the person, rather than trying to fit him or her into provision that happens to be available. The tendency to secure a place that will accommodate a set number of people and then find the desired number of occupants does no favour to anyone. People need the kind of housing which suits them best, living with people with whom they are compatible and in the kind of area they want to live. This can only be achieved on an individual basis. (Mental Health Foundation, 1996)

For more details about supported living see:
Kinsella, P. (1993) *Supported living: A new paradigm?*, Manchester: National Development Team

For an introduction to one model of supported living – Keyring's Living Support Networks – see:
Pavillion Publishing in association with New Era Housing Association (1996) *Front door keys: Housing opportunities for people with learning disabilities*, Brighton: Pavilion.

Commissioning services differently

The focus on group provision is an historical legacy. Its continuation is linked to the way that service provision is funded. With the separation of the commissioning and purchasing of services from provision during the 1990s local authorities were presented with an opportunity to change this.

The most common way that day service provision is funded at present is through block payments to providers to run services, in part if not in full. For independent sector providers the payment is linked to a contract with the commissioning agency. For local authority providers there may be some form of internal contracting with the commissioning arm of the parent organisation, but this is relatively underdeveloped.

Funding residential services is more complex because of the place of state benefits in the funding equation. A local authority or health authority may still make a block payment to an organisation for a set number of placements in their provision. From this would be deducted each individual's own contribution to their care costs, funded through their benefits income. The purchasing authority then seeks to fill, and keep full, the placements they have purchased. Many residential providers set their fee level at the benefits threshold for people needing lower levels of support and do not need to have a contract with a purchasing authority. In theory, their only contact could be through the registration and inspection process for residential homes.

These systems have supported organisations and services rather than people:
- Block funding has encouraged slotting people into existing services rather than identifying opportunities and support to match the person's specific requirements.
- Block funding contributes to the service's overall costs, which may include high central management overheads and the maintenance of large buildings that serve to set people apart from the community in which they live.
- Block contracts have generally not been rigorously managed in terms of comparing central organisational costs across providers and quality of life outcomes for service recipients in relation to fee levels. In some areas, where provision of some forms of support has been limited, providers have been able to dictate prices.
- Because funding has not been seen as buying identified services and support for individuals, organisations have used their staff to focus on service tasks rather than achieving outcomes for specific people.
- The emphasis on the purchasing responsibilities of care managers has led to a lack of monitoring for people whose services are not paid for from the care management budget. As a result many have languished in long-term placements that are not providing a good quality of life.
- Block funding gives service recipients little control over the opportunities and support they receive from a provider organisation.

Individualised purchasing and care management

Person-centred planning can be used by a care manager to develop a detailed specification for services – or opportunities and support – needed by an individual. A contract with a service provider can be centred on the individual service specification, and monitoring focuses on whether that specification has been met. The person's wishes and needs are at the heart of the process, and resources are focused on the individual.

Unfortunately, care management across the UK has struggled to deliver on the promise of more individualised support for people. Most care management teams have far too few workers for the number of people receiving services. They work in a pressured environment which makes it difficult to really get to know a person, their wishes and support needs. Effective monitoring becomes impossible. Unless the number of care managers is increased countrywide the onus will be on the provider services and people's informal support networks to ensure that individuals get opportunities and support that is right for them.

There are some things that can be done to make the system work in a more person-centred way:

- Authorities can train their commissioning and purchasing staff in person-centred planning so that they have a shared vision and common understanding of the process and the outcomes required. Involving service recipients as trainers can be a powerful tool.
- Commissioners can use their contracts with service providers to ensure that person-centred planning is carried out, and then use the information as the basis for regular monitoring of a person's support package by a care manager. Resources would need to be identified to support the person-centred planning process.
- Care management teams can organise themselves in different ways to ensure that people who have been using services for many years start to receive regular monitoring. This can help people move on from residential homes and day centres that are not offering the life opportunities they want, and also help those services to change. The London Borough of Hackney attached named care managers to day centres and hostels to ensure that the needs and wishes of the people in those services were identified and person-centred plans drawn up. Other authorities have set up separate teams to focus on monitoring people's support packages.
- Commissioners can deliberately develop services that provide more individualised support by drawing up a detailed specification that requires the service to develop natural supports for people. An example of one such specification is shown in the **Appendix**. An issue for care managers is that when they want to purchase support for people to do specific things they often have to resort to bringing in agency workers because there are no local options. They are then drawn into directly managing and supervising the worker on the specific task – which often proves impossible. Commissioners need to 'manage the market' and develop a range of support options.

Attaching funding to individuals means that if the person moves on then the funding moves with them. It creates greater flexibility and real options, and makes it easier to get people the right opportunities and support.

Direct payments

Attaching the funding through a direct payment to the person goes a step further by placing control of the money in the hands of that individual (with support from others if needed). The Independent Living Fund has followed this approach for many years and disabled people have successfully led independent lives as a result.

Swindon People First got fed up with waiting for their local authority to introduce a Direct Payment scheme so did it themselves! With funding from Comic Relief they have set up their own scheme.

See: People First (1999a) 'Moving on with Direct Payments', *Community Living*, Oct/Nov.

The person becomes the purchaser of their own support and controls it. It is important to give people support to manage a direct payment if they need it. Those commissioning and contracting a support scheme have to find ways of ensuring that people are themselves in the driving seat. Such support has been provided to people through Independent Living Centres, Service Brokerage Schemes and Independent Advocacy Schemes. Independence from the funding organisation is a key requirement.

For more information on direct payments see:
> Holman, A. and Bewley, C. (1999) *Funding freedom 2000 – People with learning difficulties using Direct Payments*, VIA.
> DoH (2000) *The easy guide to Direct Payments*, London: DoH (available as CD, tape or booklet).

Direct payments may be particularly helpful for people from minority ethnic groups who wish to ensure that they are supported by someone who shares their culture.

Many local authority commissioners still need to make direct payments a real option for people by putting support schemes in place.

Developing better local support options

In many areas day centres and residential homes still predominate. There is little employment support available and access to well-supervised and managed individual support is limited. The onus is on commissioners to change that picture.

One option is to simply tell providers that they have to change the way they do things, and paint a clear picture of what's wanted, tying it into the contract review and renewal process; another is to look for other providers who may be able to create what's wanted from scratch through retendering of the resources tied up in that service; another is to change the way that funding is allocated to the service and attach it to individuals. All of these approaches have drawbacks.

- Telling providers they have to change but not giving them active leadership or support to do so is unlikely to lead to the development of what commissioners really want. These are complex organisational changes that can feel daunting and risky. Providers need to know that there is a joint investment; that they are doing it in partnership with the commissioners and will have help solving problems along the way.

- Looking to other providers to develop a new service at the expense of an existing one usually means that service recipients have little say in the development process. People may be indicating that they want other opportunities but closing the service entirely is unlikely to be their chosen option. People will be particularly concerned about friendships and bonds they have built up with each other and with staff.

- Individualised funding can be seen as a threat to the stability and long-term viability of a service because core costs are met through the sum total of individual contracts. If the number of individual contracts reduce, cash-flow problems may result, affecting service delivery and viability. Organisations are less likely to invest in expenditure that actually helps to improve and develop provision – like training for staff, team development, new initiatives – unless they have some core financial confidence and stability.

Provider organisations need help to get from where they are now to the different forms of provision explored earlier. This means commissioners working in partnership with them and nurturing their development. This may involve difficult negotiating and straight talking to reach an agreed plan. It can help if the service's funding is changed so that it is more focused on individuals but also meets concerns about core costs and development costs. This can be achieved through a small core contract supported by individual contracts for every service recipient. Creative thinking and a 'let's try it' approach are important qualities for commissioners.

Monitoring

Chapter 5 describes how JRHT residents were involved in monitoring the quality of opportunities and support people were getting. This is one way that commissioners can ensure that services become more person-centred.

In the London Borough of Newham people with learning difficulties monitor the quality of local residential homes. They prepare a report for the 'buyers' (the commissioners) which helps to ensure that the provision meets the standards that service recipients want. The 'Quality Network' – a project led by the National Development Team and British Institute of Learning Disabilities – is based on the same principle – that the views of people with learning difficulties about important aspects of a service should lie at the heart of monitoring.

> For more information about involving service recipients in commissioning and monitoring see:
> People First (1999b) *Putting people first: Our way to do things better*, London: People First.
> Simons, K. (1999) *A place at the table*, Kidderminster: BILD Publications.
>
> The NDT/BILD (British Institute of Learning Disabilities) Quality Network can be contacted at:
> Slade House, Horspath Driftway, Headington, Oxford OX3 7JH
> Telephone: 01865 228186
> Fax: 01865 228 173
> Website: qualitynetwork.org.uk

Monitoring the quality of life of people living in their own homes is a particularly sensitive area. National guidelines on the regulation of supported living may soon be produced for commissioners to help address the issues, but it is clear that people's family and friends already play an important role. Having a circle of support or a planning circle – a network of people looking out for a person – makes it more likely that support shortfalls will be noticed and acted on. What is needed is a clear mechanism for people to raise any day-to-day concerns, and a system for periodic reporting by people who are very involved with the person but independent of the housing and support providers.

9
A final overview

Involvement with the JRHT has provided the Changing Days project with significant learning. All the previous work was carried out within day services in the statutory sector. The Joseph Rowntree experience provided lessons from the voluntary sector, in a housing trust smaller in scale than most health or social services organisations. Helping individuals plan their lives from where they live gave insights about ordinary patterns of living that did not depend on attendance at day services. It offered time to reflect on how to make best use of the person's environment, exploring ways in which people could build relationships, and contribute to and participate more in their community.

Setting the context

The Trust's development work in their residential community homes was firmly rooted in a number of policy initiatives of the 1990s. The 1990 Community Care Act marked a significant step towards services being more focused on individuals, particularly through care management. Higher expectations around understanding and meeting individual needs, including individualising budgets, ran parallel with serious funding cuts in the statutory sector. Throughout the latter half of the 1990s, redesigning day services was held back by the difficulties of providing funding to support community-based services while at the same time running down conventional day centres, and by the lack of new monies to develop supported employment, leisure and education.

The impact of funding cuts has been strongly felt within the voluntary sector. Contractual agreements with social services have provided little or no growth to improve the quality of people's lives. This meant that when the Rowntree work started in 1998, people living in the homes were at least partially dependent on traditional day centres. Lack of individual contracts and funding resulted in people 'fitting into' existing services with little opportunity to shape their own day opportunities. A key aim, therefore, was to move towards tailor-made, individual patterns of living.

The post-institutional era

The closure of long-stay hospitals led to the development of a range of housing options for people in the community. However, the growth of individual, and often high quality, physical living environments was not matched by a growth in individual lifestyles which enabled people to become participating citizens of their local communities. In retrospect it is evident that building the community 'infrastructure' should have received equal attention along with the 'bricks and mortar' of resettlement.

The need to tackle the social exclusion of disabled people and people with learning difficulties was a key factor in setting up the Changing Days project, including the work with the Joseph Rowntree Foundation. The advantages of working within the voluntary sector came to light as the project discovered the greater flexibility in decision making, a less formal hierarchy and less complex systems of change. People living in the homes seemed to have a real identity within the organisation and were known as individuals by senior and middle managers as well as front-line staff. The smaller scale organisation offered a more personal service.

The current policy context

Translating policy into practice which results in better lives for people has become a significant issue for all service providers. The list of policy initiatives seems never-ending and while positive and inspirational in their aims and values, they have significantly increased the workload of most managers and front line workers. The big question, and most demanding task, is how to translate policies into real services and support.

Recent policy initiatives

- *Modernising social services* (DoH, 1998b) – with emphasis on independence, social inclusion and user driven services

- *Partnership initiatives* (DoH, 1998a) – promoting work across agencies and encouraging holistic planning, provision and shared assessments

- *Signposts for success* (DoH, 1998c) and *Once a day* (NHS Executive, 1999b) – highlight the unmet healthcare needs of individuals and how to better meet them

- *Welfare to Work* (NHS Executive, 1999a) – offering more opportunities for supported and mainstream employment

- Joint Investment Plans (a practical means of planning together, across agencies, to better meet the needs of the local population)

- Health Improvement Plans (to give special focus to the healthcare needs of individuals)

There have also been significant publications such as *Facing the facts* (DoH, 1999) which talks about the limited life choices on offer to people and the lack of opportunities in the community. The report also stresses the lack of alternatives to traditional day services. Comments from residents of JRHT homes, following a consultation held early in 1995, backed up this view and was a catalyst for the setting up of the Changing Days work.

The most recent policy initiative, the National Service Framework, will aim to improve the life chances of individuals through an emphasis on creating and encouraging independence, achieving greater employment opportunities, offering more choice about where and with whom people live, and the strong promotion of social inclusion. The Framework will also emphasise the importance of involving housing, education, leisure and the benefits systems. It will outline standards that need to be achieved by all commissioners and providers.

With this policy context in mind and with a commitment to helping individuals find better day opportunities, JRHT managers and staff demonstrated that change can happen for individuals and that policy can help focus on priorities for change.

Characteristics of positive change

The experience with the JRHT has given many lessons in how to improve the quality of life of people living in community-based homes. Some of the key ingredients are:

- a clear value base owned by managers, carers, staff and people who use services;

- strong, consistent leadership that provides a framework for change, inspires people and manages the emotional turbulence of change;

- staff with skills to understand and support the unique needs of each individual, turn goals into action, and to work with ordinary members of the public;

- staff recruited specifically to help establish and support planning circles, complete person-centred plans and keep the focus on achieving change for individuals;

- an organisational environment with a flat hierarchy, an open system of communication, and a culture focused on regular positive outcomes for people;

- a capacity to manage resistance to change and sensitively address fears and concerns;

- a culture where measured risks can be taken and where imaginative and creative community-based solutions are the norm;

- a partnership with parents and carers which recognises and values everyone's role and shares planning and support for the individual;

- a partnership across all statutory services which pools funds and resources, reduces wasteful duplication and thus increases people's chances of getting good support;

- bringing service recipients together to consider common concerns, gain strength from each other and collectively voice their views about the services they receive.

The policy and value base for achieving greater community involvement and ordinary day opportunities is already rooted in the JRHT and other agencies. What remains is the challenge of supporting individuals, one person at a time, to realise their hopes and dreams. Only a continued emphasis on this value base and commitment to the hard work of putting it into practice will result in achieving the goal of social inclusion and full citizenship for all.

References and further reading

Bradley, A. (1999) *Taking turns – Around recreation and leisure*, Kidderminster: BILD Publications (3 booklets): 1. You're on [for people with learning difficulties], 2. Your turn [for parents] 3. Over to you! [for staff].

DoH (Department of Health) (1998a) *Partnership in action: new opportunities for joint working between health and social services*, London: DoH.

DoH (1998b) *Modernising social services: Promoting independence, improving protection, raising standards*, London: The Stationery Office.

DoH (1998c) *Signposts for success in commissioning and providing health services for people with learning disabilities*, London: DoH.

DoH (1999) *Facing the facts: Services for people with learning disabilities: A policy impact study of social care and health services*, London: DoH.

DoH (2000) *The easy guide to Direct Payments*, London: DoH (available as CD, audio-tape or booklet).

Emerson, E., Robertson, J., Gregory, N., Hatton, C., Kessissogglou, S., Hallam, A., Knapp, M., Järbnsk, K., Netter, P. and Noonan Walsh, P. (1999) *Quality and costs of residential supports for people with learning disabilities*, Manchester: Hester Adrian Research Centre.

English National Board for Nursing, Midwifery and Health Visiting (1997) *Making it happen: Community leisure and recreation for people with profound learning and multiple disabilities*, London: ENB.

Felce, D. (1996) 'Quality of support for ordinary living', in J. Mansell and K. Ericsson (eds) *Deinstitutionalisation and community living: Intellectual disability services in Britain, Scandinavia and the USA*, London: Chapman and Hall.

Grove, B. et al (1997) *The social firms handbook*, Brighton: Pavilion.

Holman, A and Bewley, C. (1999) *Funding freedom 2000 – People with learning difficulties using Direct Payments*, VIA.

Kinsella, P. (1993) *Supported living: A new paradigm?*, Manchester: National Development Team.

McIntosh, B. and Whittaker, A. (eds) (1998) *Days of change. A practical guide to developing better day opportunities with people with learning difficulties*, London: King's Fund.

McIntosh, B. and Whittaker, A. (eds) (2000) *Unlocking the future. Developing new lifestyles with people who have complex disabilities*, London: King's Fund.

Mental Health Foundation (1996) *Building expectations: Opportunities and services for people with a learning disability*, London: Mental Health Foundation.

Mount, B., Ducharme, G. and Beeman, P. (1991) *Person-centred development: A journey in learning to listen to people with disabilities*, Manchester, CT: Communitas.

Netten, A. and Dennett, J. (1997) *Unit costs of health and social care*, Canterbury: PSSRU, University of Kent

NHS Executive (1999a) *Welfare to work: New deal in the NHS*, (HSC 1999/225), London: DoH.

NHS Executive (1999b) *Once a day: One or more people with learning disabilities are likely to be in contact with your primary healthcare team – how can you help them?*, London: DoH.

O'Brien, J. (1987) 'A guide to personal futures planning', in T.G. Bellamy and B. Wilcox (eds) *A comprehensive guide to the activities catalogue. An alternative curriculum for youths and adults with severe disabilities*, Baltimore MD: Paul H Brookes.

Pavilion Publishing (1987) *Participation in everyday activities, Bringing People Back Home Series*, Brighton: Pavillion Publishing.

Pavillion Publishing in association with New Era Housing Assoaciation (1996) *Front door keys: Housing opportunities for people with learning disabilities*, Brighton: Pavillion.

Pearpoint, J., O'Brien, J. and Forest, M. (1993) PATH (Planning Alternative Tomorrows with Hope) *A workbook for planning possible positive futures*, Toronto, Canada: Inclusion Press.

People First (1999a) 'Moving on with Direct Payments', *Community Living*, Oct/Nov.

People First (1999b) *Putting people first: Our way to do things better*, People First.

Sanderson, H., Kennedy, J., Ritchie, P. and Goodwin, G. (1997) *People, plans and possibilities: Exploring person-centred planning*, Scotland: SHS Ltd.

Simons, K. (1998) *Home, work and inclusion: The social policy implications of supported living and employment for people with learning disabilities*, York: Joseph Rowntree Foundation.

Simons, K. (1999) *A place at the table*, Kidderminster: BILD Publications.

Smull, M. and Harrison, S.B. (1992) *Supporting people with severe reputations in the community*, Alexandria VA: National Association of State Directors of Developmental Disabilities Inc.

Turner, C. (1995) *The Eureka principle*, Shaftesbury: Element.

Wertheimer, A. (ed) (1995) *Circles of support: Building inclusive communities*, Bristol: Circles Network.

Wertheimer, A. (ed) (1996) *Changing days: Developing new day opportunities with people who have learning difficulties*, London: King's Fund.

Whittaker, A. (1999) *Changing our days: Finding ways to get what you want from life*, (Book and audio compact disc), London: King's Fund.

Appendix: Specification for a personal assistant scheme for people with learning difficulties

Who is the scheme for?

Adults with learning difficulties who are the financial responsibility of the Borough and who need assistance with at least **two** of the following:

- physically moving from place to place (eg, from wheelchair to a toilet)
- intimate personal care (eg, going to the toilet, dealing with soiled underwear, etc)
- eating and drinking (ie, without support they wouldn't eat or drink)
- preventing self-harm or harm to others.

The scheme focuses on people who need a very high level of assistance due to additional physical and/or sensory disabilities and/or behaviours that may lead to harm.

Where and when would the assistance take place?

This is *not* a home-based personal assistant scheme. The scheme is about assisting people when away from their homes. The person may be participating in group activities or undertaking an activity on their own. It is likely that most activities will be during the day, although a few may be in the evenings or at weekends.

People could be undertaking activities in a range of different places during the week. Some may be doing things away from home five days a week, others only two or three.

Assisting people to do what?

The scheme is *not* just about assisting people with the daily living activities listed above. It is also about helping people with multiple disabilities to lead more ordinary lives and take part in a range of different opportunities and activities. They will require help *to actually take part* (in whatever way they can) in the activity of their choice.

The personal assistant is there *for the person*. He or she needs to get to know the person and assist them to take as much control as possible over their own life. It is an active role, focused on one person, which will require sensitivity to the changing wishes and needs of the person.

What the person does on a day-to-day basis will have been agreed as part of their individual plan.

Requirements

The scheme must:
- Be focused on individuals and be responsive to their specific needs and preferences.
- Draw on and use the knowledge that exists about individuals in their current support network.
- Involve the people being assisted, their family carers and advocates, and give them as much control as possible within the scheme.
- Assist people to 'get their voice heard' on a daily basis.
- Be able to respond to the differing requirements of individuals in relation to their gender, culture, ethnicity and age.
- Demonstrate a commitment to assisting people to access new opportunities.
- Work to, and achieve high standards of practice, and be able to demonstrate this.
- Provide consistent and reliable assistance to individuals.
- Be a safe place for the individuals who are receiving assistance.
- Have adequate support, supervision, training, monitoring and management for its staff.
- Support its staff to work effectively alongside staff employed by other service providers.
- Be able to respond flexibly to meet increased demand or new ways of working in the future.
- Present good value for money.

Organisations bidding to run the scheme need to show:

- What you will do to meet the requirements listed above (with supporting examples of any similar activities that are already being done in your existing service provision).
- How the scheme would be structured, and how it would actually operate day to day.
- How the short lead-in time for the development would be addressed.
- The hours of assistance per week that could be purchased with £120,000 annually, with a breakdown of staffing costs, contingency costs, management and running costs, and an overall unit cost per hour of assistance.

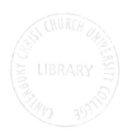